Intermittent Fasting 101

A complete guide to unlock your weight loss potential and live a healthier life for women: quick recipe ideas and 16 effective lifestyle methods to achieve the best results!

[Felicia Sanders]

Table of Contents

Your notes

Your notes

INTRODUCTION

Within the past few years, the concept of Intermittent Fasting has started to trend heavily, impacting anyone interested in dieting and healthy living. Its origins, however, are much more ancient than most of us would ever think. In this chapter, you'll be introduced to the long history of Intermittent Fasting so that you can better understand how that trajectory leads to today. By the end of this section, you should feel confident that you know where the tradition came from, as well as what it has to do with you—reading this book in this very moment.

IF for Primitive Humans

Intermittent Fasting has been a practice as long as humans have existed. In the times of our most primitive ancestors, IF wasn't so much a chosen lifestyle as it was a necessity. It came down to the prevalence and availability of food—and the hunter's and gatherer's abilities to acquire it.

In these ancient times, people would have had to go longer between meals and sometimes perhaps spend days without eating. However, what arose from necessity produced incredible and even sustainable physical, mental, and emotional effects. These ancient people would have also (likely unintentionally) been able to concentrate better, live longer, slowing age and digest with ease consistently.

Primitive humans would also occasionally fast for shared purposes once societies and civilizations started assembling. For instance, before going off to war, communities would fast, and young people coming-of-age would fast as part of those rituals. Sometimes societies would also demand a fast as an offering to the gods or to implore the end of natural disasters such as floods or famines.

Religious Instances of IF

On the same vein as using a fast as an offering to the gods, many ancient cultures eventually required some fasting for their religion purposes. Consider Christianity. Orthodox Christians of the Greek variety still practice their ancient fasts, which comprise almost 200 days out of the year. Non-Orthodox Christians are also invited to fast whenever moved to do so to become closer to the Holy Trinity.

Consider Buddhism. The practice of intermittent fasting has always been essential to reaching enlightenment, because it helps the soul undo its ropes to the body. The enlightened one, Siddhartha, practiced fasting for many years as a method to acquire wisdom.

Consider Judaism. The day before Passover, it is an ancient tradition followed still today that the first-born child of each family should fast to celebrate the miracle from Moses' time that spared all Hebrew first-borns. Furthermore, Jewish people are invited to fast throughout the year at any point to celebrate a life lost, to appeal to God or a prophet, or to express sorrow for a sin or wrong committed.

Consider Islam. The holy month of Ramadan features a 4-week-long fast from the time the sun rises to the time the sun sets. During this time, drinks are also shunned, as well as alcohol drinking, smoking, or performing any bad habits or repetitive practices that don't serve the soul. Muhammad, the prophet of Islam, also suggested his followers fast every Monday and Thursday (essentially the 5:2 method), but it's unclear how consistently this suggestion is heeded.

Other religions across the world have also required a temporary fast for spiritual reasons, and it is true that many have gotten closer to their gods through this practice. However, there are so many more benefits to fasting than just these spiritual ones, and these other applications are made clear in the next chapters.

From the Past to Now

On top of being used for survival and religious purposes, intermittent fasting has gained appeal through time for its medical applications as well. Even millennia before its trending popularity today, back in 400 BC, intermittent fasting made an appearance and gained popularity by the suggestion of Hippocrates.

Yes, that Hippocrates! The infamous "father of modern medicine" advocated for fasting to heal almost any internal injury or state of disease. He once wrote, "To eat when you are sick, is to feed your illness," if that gives you any indication of the incredible uses he found for the practice.

Other ancient Greek philosophers, writers, and historians have echoed these concepts from Hippocrates through time into the early years, AD. Essentially, just like how animals seem to "fast" when they're getting sick or feeling unwell, humans have the same instincts but often ignore them, pushing through the illness and feeding it with food when the body needs the exact opposite.

Past the ancient Greeks, however, other thinkers across time have affirmed the same feelings. For example, Paracelsus (another founder of modern medicine) famously wrote, "Fasting is the greatest remedy," and Benjamin Franklin (one of America's founding fathers) also once inscribed in a journal, "The best of all medicines is resting and fasting."

In the past, fasting has also been used as a form of political protest, and the most famous instance of this happening occurred with Mahatma Gandhi, who lasted 21 days at his longest period of fasting. His goals were to protest against India's dependence on Britain and to acquire freedom and integrity for his people. Many others have taken up fasting for similar aims, but none have been so successful or so famous, it seems.

Contemporary Applications

Now, it seems that fasting has gained new fame in the form of Intermittent Fasting, and the capital letters here are used intentionally to connote the almost "patented" application of these ancient theories in relation to health and weight loss in recent times.

This practice of Intermittent Fasting has been trending for the past few years, and its impact has spread widely since then. People have lost incredible amounts of weight. They've seen their energy levels improve drastically. They've been able to heal brain disorders and reverse the signs of ageing. People across the world have come to understand what amazing uses fasting can have, and they are becoming healthier because of these realisations.

Doctors who have practiced fasting cures for decades have almost consistently welcomed the increased interest in IF these days, for they know how much good this practice can do for so many. Fasting is still used for religious and spiritual purposes, and some still practice it as they strive to survive. For others, IF today is revered as the so-called "fountain of youth," and many dietary plans are starting to incorporate its themes.

Overall, it seems that IF has been used throughout time for three main things: survival, spiritual connection, and body/mind health. These applications are valid today, but the focus tends toward that final point in the list: body/mind health. For those seeking a state of internal balance, IF can be a blessing. For those intrigued by IF, keep reading to find out more and to learn how to build this practice into your daily routine.

CHAPTER 1: WHAT IS INTERMITTENT FASTING?

The Science Behind Intermittent Fasting

Understanding how exactly intermittent fasting work is one of the essential elements that need to be covered before you dive into it and start adopting this method of eating in your own life. By learning more about how it works, you can get a better idea of whether or not this might be a good option for you – and if you would be able to benefit from it truly.

This eating habit basically involves cycles of eating and abstaining from food. There are different techniques and methods that have been introduced over the last few years, so not everyone will follow this lifestyle option in the same way as others. Generally, however, all options that are available involved periods of time where food is consumed, and then periods where the person would completely avoid eating any type of food.

When eating normally, with three meals a day and in-between snacks, the body uses energy from the recently consumed meal first, seeking out carbohydrates (CHO) and sugars, which it prefers to burn before anything else. Without intermittent fasting, normal persons (non-diabetics) insulin sensitivity will be at normal levels, and will detect stored glycogen at "full level." With sufficient blood glucose levels, excess energy will be stored as fat. If this happens on a regular basis, the determinants for the difference in body weight will lie in the level of activity and metabolic rate which slows down with age, resulting in weight gain.

When on intermittent fasting, the body behaves differently when food is present (feasting) and during the period of abstinence (fasting), as compared to normal eating. The body produces insulin in response to the presence of food, enabling the body to get the most from them, maximising nutrients for optimum results. Since eating is confined to a desired set window of 4, 6, or 8 hours, the body will not have a ready source of energy during the fasted state and will tend to extract energy from stored fat rather than from glucose traveling in the blood or glycogen stored in the liver or muscles.

Insulin sensitivity is increased after a fast. We can illustrate this insulin sensitivity by analysing the cascade of events that take place when such a person eats something. As blood glucose rises, it activates a feedback mechanism which signals the pancreas to send insulin to the site where it is needed. An immediate response serves to lower the blood glucose and prevent its accumulation in the blood, or hyperglycemia. Here, insulin responds with a "now you see it, now you don't" type of mechanism: a sharp peak in response to the rising blood glucose, followed by an immediate decline. This is documented by lower readings of 2-hour postprandial blood glucose and insulin measurements.

Diabetics, on the other hand, suffer from insulin resistance, wherein the pancreas secretes only small bursts of insulin in response to glucose, followed by a slowed decline, resulting in higher 2-hour postprandial blood glucose and insulin measurements.

Intermittent fasting is a weight loss diet regimen that has recently gained mainstream popularity. This fitness trend incorporates a regimen with alternate eating and fasting. Much research has focused on this diet plan. The research shows that IF helps protect the body from various diseases, enhances metabolic health, helps with weight loss, and promotes a longer life. This section will discuss what intermittent fasting is and why it is significant.

Intermittent Fasting – An Insight

This fasting method involves a cyclic pattern between fasting and eating. There is no standard rule about what to eat, but the plan does target when you have your meals. Many IF methods exist, all of which split the eating and fasting periods by days or weeks.

When you are sleeping, you are fasting. However, through intermittent fasting, that fasting period is extended for a longer duration. You can fast by not having your breakfast when you wake up and by consuming your first meal of the day at noon. Later, you can have your last meal at around 8 p.m. That way, you are fasting for almost 16 hours daily while avoiding eating for over eight hours per day. This popular method of IF is called the 16/8 technique.

It may sound complicated, but intermittent fasting is much easier to handle than other weight loss diets, such as the Ketogenic diet. Moreover, reports suggest that practitioners of this diet plan are more energetic during their fasting periods. It may be uncomfortable in the beginning, when your body adjusts to the sudden hunger cravings. However, with time, it all becomes easier and the body adapts to those hunger periods.

While you cannot eat anything during your fasting time, you can drink a non-caloric beverage, like water, black tea, or coffee. Many types of intermittent fasting regimens allow you to consume small amounts of foods that are low in calories while you are fasting. However, this technique involves a targeted approach toward meeting your goals. You can take supplements during the fasting time, but the products should not contain calories

What Is the Purpose of Fasting?

For many centuries, people have fasted. Often, fasting was done because there was no food available to consume. In other situations, it was part of a religious belief. Moreover, many animals, including humans, fast when they fall sick. Thus, fasting is a standard process, as the body can handle extended periods of time without eating anything.

However, with fasting, there are specific changes in the body so that the body can counter the lack of nutrition in that particular fasting period. This is linked to cellular repair operations, genes, and hormones. During fasting, there is a significant decrease in insulin and blood sugar levels, and a radical elevation in growth hormones.

Thus, many people practice intermittent fasting to promote weight loss, as it is one of the simplest techniques to burn fat and restrict calories. Many also follow such techniques to improve their metabolism, as fasting can regulate various health markers and risk factors. In addition, intermittent fasting has been noted to help an individual live for a longer time. This has been proven through research conducted upon rodents, which had extended lifespans after a restriction in their calorie intake.

Another prominent benefit of IF is that it can help protect the body from diseases, such as Alzheimer's disease, cancer, type 2 diabetes, heart disease, etc. Many people who practice this fasting technique do it to lose weight and do not realize that it is also benefitting them clinically.

Thus, you can consider intermittent fasting to be an essential process for regulating your body weight and health simultaneously. With fewer meals, you have a better chance of living a healthy life. In addition, when you do not have to prepare extra dishes every day (because you are skipping meals), you can save a lot of time for other activities.

CHAPTER 2: BENEFITS OF INTERMITTENT FASTING

A number of studies, like those mentioned above, have been done on both humans and animals. These studies evaluated the many benefits of intermittent fasting for controlling weight and other bodily functions. The results have been phenomenal.

Some of the popular health benefits of the IF regimen are:

- Weight loss: This is the most common health benefit that you can achieve through the intermittent fasting method. You can reduce your belly fat and weight without compromising the calorie intake.

- Insulin resistance: IF is also capable of decreasing insulin resistance in the body. A follower of this fasting technique will witness a decrease in the levels of insulin by an impressive 20 to 31%. Furthermore, IF reduces the blood sugar levels up to 6%. These figures are enough to protect a person from type 2 diabetes.

- Inflammation: Much research has revealed a decrease in inflammation markers, which have been noted to be significant catalysts for several chronic diseases.

- Cardiovascular health: IF is known to decrease bad cholesterol levels (LDL) and promote HDL or good cholesterol. In addition, it may decrease the presence of blood triglycerides, which is one of the causes of cardiovascular diseases.

- Cancer: Animals on the IF diet have shown results that display cancer prevention abilities.

- Brain function: IF improves brain function by promoting the growth of nerve cells. Thus, it can help protect against neural disorders, such as Alzheimer's disease.

- Anti-aging properties: IF has been noted to promote longevity in rats, which were part of a fasting experiment. It was found that rats following this diet lived up to 83% longer than rats that weren't on the diet.

Note that while IF may have health benefits, the experiments are still at an initial stage. Several of these studies were conducted for a short duration upon various animals. Therefore, there are still many unanswered questions.

Impact of Intermittent Fasting on Lifestyle

While eating healthy is a simple process, it is not as easy as it seems. One of its primary hurdles is the work needed to cook healthy recipes. However, it does save time by reducing the workload required to prepare several meals a day, thus letting you spend your time doing other things. This makes IF a popular choice among people who prefer life hacks to make their lives easier and healthier. In this way, IF has a significant impact on the lifestyle of an individual.

Intermittent Fasting: Mental Advantages

In addition to physical benefits, IF has mental benefits. This diet plan offers significant benefits related to:

- Boosting memory

- Shielding the mind from neurological disorders such as epilepsy and Alzheimer's disease

- Improving mental focus and clarity

Intermittent Fasting: Enhancing Cognitive Function and Reducing

Stress

Intermittent fasting has also shown significant effects with respect to the brain and memory. People who have practiced this diet plan were better able to retain their ability to learn, decreased their oxidative stress, and enhanced their memory.

Many researchers say that this activity takes place because this fasting program manipulates the brain cells to perform more efficiently. During fasting, the cells undergo low/moderate stress, which is why the most efficient cells among them start improvising and adapting to the new condition. This way, the weak cells die, but the stronger ones survive and improve the abilities of the brain.

You can compare it to a high-intensity workout routine at the gym. Exercising is also a type of physical stress that forces your body to endure uncomfortable conditions. As you progress with the regimen, your body starts to adapt to the new conditions, building your muscles, stamina, etc. However, you must rest between your workouts to keep your body ready for the next session.

A similar approach exists when you are practicing IF. Here, your resting intervals will comprise healthy and regular eating sessions, balanced with fasting sessions. That way, you can benefit both your mind and your body.

Thus, you can see that intermittent fasting is capable of improving your cognitive operations due to moderate stress at a cellular level to support and sculpt you.

Additional Benefits of Intermittent Fasting

If you are planning to try intermittent fasting, you will experience the following benefits. Remember that these results will come about only when you are following a strict fasting and eating regimen. IF will help your body achieve the following benefits:

- Improves fat loss

If you follow the 16/8 method in which you eat within an eight-hour period and fast for the remaining 16 hours, you can lose a significant amount of weight without having to worry about calories. No doubt, this method will cause the body to lose weight, but those who follow a healthy diet will be able to achieve two times the weight loss twice than those who prefer junk food achieve. Thus, through intermittent fasting, you have a way to accomplish your goals, but only when you follow it healthily.

- Increases muscle mass

Many people believe that their muscles will fade away while fasting. However, as per research, a 24-hour fast elevated the growth hormone in humans (HGH) up to 1300% for women and 2000% for men. HGH is known for its significance in building muscle cells. With such high numbers, there is a huge effect on the physique of an individual following IF. Increased HGH levels offer enhanced bone mass, increased body mass, and reduced body fat.

- Faster recovery

Increased HGH also helps synthesise protein that causes the body to repair and heal faster after an injury or workout session.

- Adds suppleness to the skin

With an increase in age, HGH levels decrease. However, during a study, participants who were provided with HGH supplements were found to build muscle and lose fat at a much higher rate. In addition, their skin improved in strength, making it more resistant to wrinkles and sagging.

- Reduces the rate of ageing

With fasting, your body starts producing stem cells at a much faster rate. These stem cells can be manipulated to become any cell in the body. Therefore, they can replace damaged and old cells, keeping your body younger at the cellular level. These stem cells can help with chronic pain, old injuries, joints, skin, etc. Therefore, instead of going for stem cell therapy, which can be costly, your other option is to focus on intermittent fasting.

- Enhances brain functions

Through fasting, you can improve your brain. When you fast, your brain starts generating a protein known as BNF, which is a very crucial building block. This protein helps improve memory and learning power.

In addition, it helps develop complex and robust neural networks to keep the brain functioning smoothly and speedily. This is necessary to keep the brain functions active as you get older.

- Triggers autophagy

This process may sound cruel for the cells in your body, but it is of crucial importance. New and strong cells eat away damaged and old cells to make space for fresh and strong ones. This is like a tune-up operation for your body; it will keep the body running smoothly and promote longevity. Through intermittent fasting, the process of autophagy can be triggered.

- Reduces inflammation

IF reduces inflammation markers and oxidative stress. Inflammation is responsible for diseases, aging, and poor performance of the body, which is why it must be reduced or eliminated. Preventing inflammation will help the body function more efficiently with increased longevity. IF offers you an upgrade that helps your body adapt to new and tougher conditions, ultimately enhancing your resistance and endurance for your eating habits. The result is a stronger, more efficient body that works on less energy.

CHAPTER 3: THE SCIENCE BEHIND

Let us start by taking a look at what intermittent fasting is. The term has become quite popular in recent years, but there is still a lot of confusion in regards to what this term really means and what it involves. Many people think that the term "intermittent fasting" refers to a diet, but this not actually a diet. Instead, it is rather an eating habit that people adopt that gives them guidance on when they should eat – this allows the digestive system to take a break from processing and digesting food continuously.

For many people, this type of dietary habit seems unhealthy. There is a lot of people who are scared of adopting this pattern of eating because they think that they would starve themselves. This, however, is a common myth that has been told about intermittent fasting.

This particular dietary scheduling technique has been used since ancient times. Numerous scientific studies have been conducted to determine how the technique interacts with the human body, and several advantages have already been noted.

An important fact that you should know when it comes to discussing this method of eating is that, since it is not classified as a diet, it will not decide the types of food that you will be eating. It is up to you to decide what you want to eat. A healthy, balanced diet that is filled with foods high in essential nutrients will, of course, result in more benefits as compared to stuffing yourself with hamburgers and pizza as soon as the clock strikes five, or whatever time it is your eating cycle starts. When opting for fast foods and other food options that are very high in carbohydrates, weight loss may not be a particular benefit that you experience when following this diet.

Why Do People Use Intermittent Fasting?

There are many different reasons why people use the intermittent fasting technique. These techniques date back to ancient times – they were used historically for a number of different purposes. For example, in older times, when a village would be limited to their food supply, people in the village would often implementing a type of fasting technique to help make the food last longer. Careful planning had to go into such a technique as the villagers had to eat enough food to support their bodily functions, at the right times, while still ensuring the inventory of available food could last until more food would become available.

Certain religions also have certain celebrations and festivals where people fast. ***Religions that incorporate fasting*** include Buddhism, Judaism, Islam, Hinduism, Bahai, Jainism, Realism, and Sikhism. Certain types of Christian religions also use fasting for various purposes. This includes Catholicism, Orthodoxy, Mormonism, and Protestantism. These religions use fasting in different ways, and the technique serves a different purpose in each religion. Some religions also only utilize parts of these fasting techniques and will not completely eliminate all foods from a person's diet for a set period of time.

Many people also tend to go on a fast when they feel sick, whether they have contracted the flu or another type of disease. This is because food does not work well with nausea and vomiting, nor with other types of gastrointestinal symptoms.

1. Blood Sugar Control by Reducing Insulin Resistance

A 24-hour Lent, without excessive exercise, lowers glycogen storage in the liver by almost 60%, so that the stored carbohydrates can easily maintain the blood sugar at a sufficient level. After 24 hours of fasting, the blood sugar level does not reach a pathological level (hypoglycemia). Also, the body can at any time through the process of gluconeogenesis produce sugar from amino acids and rely on ketones as a source of energy for the nervous system. However, this is unlikely as muscle breakdown in intermittent fasting is lower than in other diets, suggesting a muscle-sparing effect.

In modern times, however, more-and-more people are starting to adopt an intermittent fasting lifestyle – often not because they are sick or because of religious requirements, but rather due to the health benefits that have been associated with this scheduled eating habit.

While weight loss is surely the most popular benefit that tends to be the reason why people usually opt for intermittent fasting, it is important to realise that there are *more benefits* that can be achieved as well. In particular, it has been found that this technique actually changes certain cells in the body. This, in turn, can cause changes in human growth hormone regulation, insulin regulation, and even improve the body's ability to repair cells.

Fasting has also been linked to reductions in low-grade chronic inflammation throughout the body, lower levels of oxidative stress in body tissues and cells, as well as potential improvements in a person's cardiovascular health. In turn, this combination of powerful benefits may lead to a longer lifespan – while this has not been proven yet, long-term studies are currently being conducted to see whether these benefits can, in fact, prolong a person's life.

2. Enhance Heart Health by Improving Blood Pressure, Triglycerides and Cholesterol Levels

In one study, intermittent fasting in non-obese participants resulted in an increase in good HDL cholesterol in women and a reduction in triglyceride levels in men. This effect occurred over 22 days in which every two days fasted. This change may have been caused by the degradation of body fat, which was -4%.

In the case of obese people, the values improved more clearly by an average weight loss of -5.6 kg after eight weeks of alternating fasting.

Total cholesterol dropped by 21%, LDL cholesterol by 25% and triglycerides by 32% while HDL cholesterol remained unchanged.

The systolic blood pressure dropped from 124 to 116 mmHg.

Stress resistance induced by intermittent fasting has a cardio protective effect beyond reducing body weight. Studies in mice show that in a heart attack, the affected tissue in the heart is half-smaller in alternately fasting mice than in normally fed animals. Also, in cardiac infarction, 4 times fewer cardiocytes die (heart muscle cells), when the animals were fed intermittently.

3. Fighting inflammation could delay ageing and increase longevity

Both calorie restriction and intermittent fasting affect neuronal functionality, which decreases with age.

With advancing age, the so-called spine processes, which are located at the dendrites (branched cell processes) of neurons (nerve cells), decrease. The spine processes play an important role in the information transfer between the nerve cells. In rats, the number of thorns decreased by 38% after 24 months of a normal diet. Intermittent fasting prevented the reduction of the density of the spine so that rats showed little difference to 6-month-old rats even after 24 months.

Calorie reduction by the intermittent fasting increased neurogenesis (formation of new brain cells), protected the neurons from dying and stimulated the production of BDNF (brain-derived neurotrophic factor), a protein associated with increased neurogenesis, in this way, if counteracts the deterioration of the ageing process and improves the learning ability of older mice.

The effect on neurogenesis also appears to promote healing and functional recovery of spinal cord injuries in animals, whether intermittent fasting was introduced before or shortly after injury.

4. Increases Growth Hormone Secretion, Which Is Vital for Growth, Metabolism, Weight Loss and Muscle Strength, may Boost Brain Function and Prevent Neurodegenerative Disorders

Calorie restriction can have a positive effect on health and life expectancy. Some intermittent fasting researchers and advocates claim that starvation is more important than actually reducing calorie intake. Because fasting is a kind of stress for the body, it could stimulate the expression of genes that perform protective tasks and theoretically bring health benefits.

Some nutritionists assume that our ancestors did not consistently have food supplies, but were instead exposed to hunger periods and periods of increased caloric intake and that their genes were shaped and adapted accordingly. Thus, an alternate availability of food would be "natural."

IF partially dissociates the positive effect of calorie reduction from the actual total intake of calories. In mice, intermittent fasting results in improved glucose control, lower insulin levels, and greater resistance to neuronal damage regardless of weight loss or calorie intake.

Even without a reduction in calories, intermittent fasting increases the concentration of the hormone adiponectin.Adiponectin increases fat burning, anti-inflammatory, anti-diabetic and has a positive influence on cardiovascular health.

Distribution of fat deposits

In mice, intermittent fasting even without a weight loss leads to a redistribution of fat deposits in the body. The fat shifts from the visceral (in the abdomen) to the subcutaneous (under the skin) body fat. This change is healthier because visceral body fat is associated with increased inflammatory levels, insulin resistance, and metabolic syndrome. Although this effect of intermittent fasting is often mentioned by advocates, clinical studies have so far failed to detect a particularly increased decrease in visceral adipose tissue in humans.

Unfortunately, most versions of intermittent fastings, such as Eat Stop Eat, do not give users a healthy dietary change. The existing eating habits and the choice of food to be maintained, the method should only be a simplification to facilitate the calorie abstinence, however, a relearning is not promoted, which makes it easy to relapse into old habits, especially in obese people. There is a risk of migration between extremes: on the one hand fasting and on the other hand food cravings paired with the choice of low-nutrient and low-fiber, but high-calorie diet.

On the other hand, intermittent fasting provides a straightforward way to lose weight and, like any other diet, works better in some people than in others, depending on preference.

Fasting over 24 hours due to calorie restriction in calorie intake overshadows the negative effects on circadian rhythms caused by intermittent fasting, which merely shifts the meal timeslots towards evening (especially warrior diet, lean gains in part).

Side Effects

Intermittent fasting is usually very well tolerated, for some users the first few days on which they starve for longer are unusual and can cause irritation, fatigue or euphoria.

A double-blind, placebo-controlled, two-day study in which participants did not know if they were receiving any caloric or calorie-free food (in gel form) could not identify any side effects related to mental performance, physical activity, sleep, and whim.

CHAPTER 4: HEALTH EFFECTS AND WHAT TO EXPECT FROM IT

While intermittent fasting is one of the most beneficial eating patterns that you can try at present, you still need to be extremely cautious before starting. Keep in mind that it is not risk-free. This makes it necessary to talk to your physician first and find out whether it is safe for you to follow this style of eating.

Also, find out if you have any health problem or complication that might cause the negative side effects, instead of rewarding benefits, of intermittent fasting to come out. It also helps to understand the most common side effects of intermittent fasting so you can study the whole approach carefully and find out how you can avoid them as much as possible.

- **Tiredness – When doing IF, there is a high risk for you to experience tiredness and grogginess, especially if you are still a beginner. Take note that in this situation, your body will also most likely run on less energy than what it is used to. Fasting might also increase your stress level and disrupt your normal sleep patterns.**

To avoid this specific side effect of intermittent fasting, it would be helpful for you to meditate or do other activities that will lower your stress levels. If you are working out on a regular basis, then consider scheduling it during your eating period. This is helpful in conserving your energy.

In addition, keep in mind that exercising while you are on the fasted state might lower your blood sugar level, which can trigger symptoms, like confusion and dizziness. It helps to be on the safe side by working out when you have already eaten.

- **Headaches – You may be dealing with headaches because your body will tend to adjust to your new eating pattern. It could be caused by dehydration so it is advisable to drink plenty of water both during your eating window and fasting period. You may also experience headaches due to a sudden drop of your blood sugar level and the release of stress hormones during the fasting period.**

The good news is that headaches usually happen only because your body is still on the adjustment stage. This means that this side effect is not permanent. Once you get used to it, you will no longer suffer from headaches.

- **Heartburn – You may also experience heartburn due to fasting. In most cases, this problem will be resolved after around a couple of months. It is necessary to visit and consult your doctor in case your heartburn does not seem to resolve on its own even after your body has adjusted to the new eating pattern.**

Heartburn is often a result of your unfamiliarity to the fasting scenario, causing your body to release stomach acids automatically at certain times. While this can cause discomfort, this only happens at the beginning of your journey so there is no need for you to worry too much about it.

- **Brain fog – This is also another common side effect of intermittent fasting, especially if your body is not yet used to the habit of not eating. This might cause your mind to try keeping up with the new routine, leading to confusion, forgetfulness, or brain fog. Once you familiarize yourself with how IF works, though, and your body has adjusted to the habit, you can expect better brain function from fasting.**

- **Diarrhea – Another unpleasant side effect of IF is diarrhea and it usually happens to those who are still beginners in fasting. There is even a higher risk for you to experience this problem if you enter the fasting period after consuming too much carbs. This problem may be associated to the significant drop in your insulin level, signaling your kidneys to get rid of excess water. This is the reason why you might experience unwanted and watery bowel movements.**

You should also remember that your body tends to lose electrolytes via bowel movements and urination. If you experience watery stools or diarrhea, then one sign that you may experience at first is low level of sodium. With that in mind, it helps to drink broth or pickle juice during those days when you are dealing with this uncomfortable and unwanted IF side effect. It also helps to add around 1-2 pinches of salt in the water you drink.

- **Insomnia and anxiety – Both these side effects may be caused by the production of adrenaline, a counter-regulatory hormone, when you begin to fast. In most cases, this effect is actually beneficial as it results in a high metabolic rate and energy level. The problem is that the energy you get from it might be too high even during those specific times when you are supposed to be sleeping.**

This can also make you feel jittery and anxious. It could be because of consuming too much coffee especially during the beginning of your fasting journey. Your anxiety also tends to worsen if you constantly worry about the effects of fasting to your health. You can resolve these side effects by sticking to proper bedtime routines, such as turning off your gadgets and electronics ninety minutes prior to your bedtime. You can also relax with the help of Epsom salt baths.

- **Bad breath – Another unpleasant and unexpected side effect of intermittent fasting is bad breath. This often happens if you already start losing weight due to fasting. This side effect is also referred to as the keto breath characterized by your tongue becoming white and a taste of acetone in your mouth. It is mainly because acetone is known as the by-product of metabolizing fatty acid.**

A lot of those who tried fasting and experienced the keto breath tend to freak out upon noticing their white tongues. They even wrongly assume that it is a result of nutrient deficiency. If this happens to you then avoid freaking out. This is actually your body's normal reaction to the fat-burning process.

As weight loss starts slowing down, you will notice a great improvement in your breath. You will also notice your tongue going back to its normal pink color. If you really feel uncomfortable with this side effect then there are some things that you can do to manage it. One is to brush your teeth as frequently as possible all throughout the day. Drinking more water and using a tongue scraper can also help.

Intermittent fasting provides numerous benefits to those who are obese, overweight, and have average weight. However, it is not appropriate for everyone, including pregnant and breastfeeding women and those who are dealing with eating disorders and certain health issues.

This is the main reason why you have to study the effects of fasting to you as soon as you begin doing it. Listen to your own body. If you notice some unwanted side effects, find out if it is because your body is just adjusting to the routine or due to more serious issues. If you are extremely worried about the negative side effects, do not hesitate to consult your doctor to ensure your safety.

CHAPTER 5: Food to include and exclude

Before you start your first fast, however, it's helpful to know what's good to eat and drink versus what hurts the cause. This chapter is dedicated to that knowledge of what's good to eat and drink when Intermittent Fasting versus what to avoid at all costs.

10 Great Foods to Eat

When you're doing IF, you'll need to eat foods that give you enough energy to last until your next breakfast, and that can be tricky if you don't know what to look out for! This section lists 10 of the best foods to incorporate in your diet when practicing IF.

1. **Avocado** is high in calories and healthy fats, so it's perfect to have as a snack or in a meal.

2. Cruciferous vegetables like cauliflower, Brussel sprouts, broccoli, and more are full of fiber and so much more!

3. Potatoes of all kinds are great to satisfy one's hunger and provide a nutritional punch.

4. Legumes and beans of all varieties contain good carbohydrates that can help lower weight without too much restriction of calories.

5. Berries contain vitamin C, flavonoids, and antioxidants that will add a lot of good to your fast.

6. Eggs of any animal are packed with protein to help you build muscle and retain energy during the fast.

7. Wild-caught fish have a great amount of protein as well as vitamin D for one's brain and healthy fats and omega-3s for one's body.

8. <u>Anything high in protein *or* high in probiotic content *will be good to have along for the ride.*</u>

9. 2.Grains and nuts are full of fiber, and healthy fats for snacks or meals during your fast's eating windows.

10. Spices such as **cayenne pepper, psyllium husk, or dried dandelion** are natural weight loss agents that can help anyone's process.

3 Foods to Avoid

On the flip side, some foods will absolutely set you back on your path to progress, and it will be equally important to know what to steer clear of. The following list includes three foods to avoid at all costs.

1. **Processed foods** will be the most important things to avoid, especially as you prepare for your fast.

2. Highly GMO foods are also things to avoid when you're working through your fast. They can offset the actual nutrition being provided by other foods in your diet.

3. ***Sugary foods*** *may curb your appetite, but they won't do anything good for your body in the long run. Steer clear for your future ease.*

10 Great Drinks

Even when you are fasting, drinks are still allowed! Make sure to choose drinks that are nutritious but not too filling, and mix it up whenever you can to keep things from getting stagnant for your taste buds (and body). 10 of the best drinks to incorporate for IF are listed below.

1. **Water with fruit or veggie slices** will provide nourishment and flavour for those times when you're fasting and need a little extra boost!

2. Probiotic drinks like kombucha or kefir will work to heal your gut and tide you over till the next eating window.

3. Black coffee will become your new best friend but be sure not to add cream and sugar! They detract from the good work coffee can do for your body during IF.

4. Teas of any kind are soothing as well as healing for various elements of the body, mind, and soul. Once again,

be sure to omit the cream and sugar!

5. Chilled or heated broths made from vegetables, bone, or animals can sustain one's energy during times of fast, too.

6. Apple Cider Vinegar shots are great for the tummy and for healing overall! Hippocrates' remedy for any ailment included this and a healthy regimen of fasting occasionally, so you're sure to succeed with this trick.

7. Water with salt can provide electrolytes, hydration, and brief sustenance for anyone whose stomachs won't stop grumbling.

8. Fresh-pressed juices are always great for the body, mind, and soul, and in times of IF, they can sustain one's energy and mood during day-long fast periods, in particular.

9. Wheatgrass shots are just as healthy as ACV shots, with a whole other subset of benefits. To awaken your body and give a jolt to your system, try these on for size.

10. **Coconut water** is more hydrating than standard water, and it's full of additional nutrients, too! Try this alternative if you need some enhancement to your usual water.

3 Drinks to Avoid

On the flip side, some drinks will definitely push you back from your goals, so keep an eye out for the 3 listed below! Avoid them at all costs.

1. **Sodas of any kind**, whether diet or non-diet, are to be avoided absolutely. They are high in sugar and riddled with terrible things for your body. Try to steer clear of this drink, especially during fast periods.

2. Coconut and almond drinks that are high in sugar are also to be avoided. Artificial sweeteners are killers for one's blood sugar and insulin levels. They will reverse all the good work you've done, so be cautious.

3. **Alcohol** will distract you from your focus and commitment to the fast, and it will also steer your body off-course from where you want it to be. Try to IF soberly.

CHAPTER 6: ADVICE FOR PREGNANT WOMEN

Fasting while pregnant might pose a danger to both mother and child, as the shortened eating window can cause weight loss. Although there is no concrete evidence that shows whether a pregnant woman should fast or not, certain studies have shown that fasting while pregnant might later affect the baby in the future. Fasting while pregnant can be detrimental to your health or your baby's health, as you both need food for survival and abstinence from food might cause a lot of havoc.

This comes into play very early in human life. Research has shown that infants born of mothers who smoked cigarettes during pregnancy may become more obese than individuals whose mum didn't smoke cigarettes. Same applies to children whose mothers had diabetes while pregnant; there's a 70% possibility that these children will become obese later in the future. Since 1980, worldwide obesity has really increased and over 1.9 billion adults were overweight, according to the World Health Organisation. The hypothalamus is a small segment of the brain which is known for regulating the intake of food. Sometimes, the storage of fat runs low; when this happens, the leptin level is forced to reduce and the appetite is then stimulated by the hypothalamus in an attempt to speed up the intake of food and also regain lost energy stores. When the levels of leptin are high, it suppresses the appetite and reduces food intake while encouraging the body to burn up extra fuel. Although leptin is an important regulator of food consumption, it cannot be used to treat obesity. Now, do all these explain why we gain weight? One of the reasons people gain weight is because they have inherited fat genes from their parents. Genetics plays a huge role in determining the physical appearance of animals, including human beings. You may be inclined to be tall, fat or short because of genetic reasons. A lot of fat people come from fat families; however, there are some people who are fat not because they are from a fat family, but because of other factors. I personally know two different people who should have been fat but ended up being thin instead. This is because other factors are responsible in determining a person's physical appearance apart from genetics.

How true is the law of thermodynamics in weight gain and weight loss? The law of thermodynamics says that "the amount of energy that goes into a machine (the human body for instance) has to balance the amount that goes out or the extra energy that goes in (food) has to be stored somehow (fat)." This simply means that no matter what your genetic variability is, lowering the food intake or increasing your energy output (exercise) will definitely reduce the energy stored as fat. It also means that eating less and less or exercising more and more will cause weight loss, according to the theory of thermodynamics.

One of the latest research studies has also shown that the modern diet has a lot of effects on people's weight. I would like to tell the story of an Indian tribe to buttress this point. There was an Indian tribe that lived in an arid part of the west. This tribe had lived there for many generations. Apparently, the land was so unproductive that none of the other tribes were ever inclined to wage war against them. They survived really well on low-calorie diets. However, when the white men arrived, bringing their own accustomed high-calorie diet with them, the Indians became really fat and over 90% of them suffered from diabetes and obesity. This only shows that the modern diet has a lot to do with why people get fat. One other reason why people get fat is sugar. Most Americans consume a massive amount of sugar every day. Instead of paying attention to calories, you will need to pay more attention to the rate at which you consume sugar. Take for instance, the whole world already knows about the calorie in calorie out thing, and when you go to stores, you find that every food item is marked low calorie. How then do people still get fat if everything is low calorie and the calories have been cut down so much? This only means that the real problem might not be calories. Research has also shown that those who eliminate sugar in their diet tend to lose more weight than those who count calories, and this same research also showed that this set of people is healthier than those who count calories.

One other ridiculous reason why you may get fat is that you are always late, although a lot of people would find this ridiculous and raise an eyebrow. However, the truth is that if you are one of those people who are always running behind schedule, it means you might be a victim of stress, which only results in the release of the stress hormone called cortisol, having been shown to cause headaches, distress, high blood pressure and of course, a slower metabolism. To crown it all, the kind of food you crave when stressed out happens to be fatty or sugar-laden food. One other cause of weight gain people do not really pay attention to is the aftermath of dehydration. Some people who are always dehydrated respond to thirst wrongly, as they eat while thirsty. Eating every time you get thirsty only does more harm than good for your health and especially your weight, instead of drinking water.

CHAPTER 7: HOW TO START GETTING RESULTS

Once you have consulted a certified nutritionist or your doctor and you gained their approval for trying intermittent fasting then you have to arm yourself with the right knowledge about how it works so you can use it to your best advantage. So how can you really maximise the benefits of intermittent fasting? Adapt it while keeping in mind these tips:

Start small and in a slow and simple manner

Intermittent fasting takes a lot of discipline and getting used to, so you should avoid rushing into the process. Start small and do it on a simple and gradual manner. Choose to do one small and simple thing related to IF to begin with. For instance, you can start by making adjustments on your regular meal schedules by 1-2 hours. There is no need to do a drastic change right away. Find out if the adjustment works and slowly work towards following your preferred IF method.

You also need to get to know more about yourself first. Spend time carefully observing your own experiences. Prior to starting, it is necessary to gather as much data and insights as possible. The information you gathered will help you in drawing conclusions that you will find useful in executing your future action once you start the IF approach. Just remember to take your time. In fact, some spent several weeks before they finally mastered the new program and made it a part of their lifestyle.

Determine the results you want to achieve

Avoid starting intermittent fasting if you do not have a clear idea about the results you wish to achieve. Know exactly what you want to gain from practicing IF. By knowing your preferred outcome, you get the chance to pick the most suitable IF method for you.

You can try intermittent fasting if you wish to delve deeper into the physical and psychological experiences associated with hunger. Intermittent fasting is also the right approach if you wish to attain the following results:

- **Learn to distinguish between actual hunger and simple cravings**

- Let go of your fear of hunger

- Improve sensitivity to insulin

- Recalibrate the use of stored fuel within your body

- Understand the eating process and respect the privilege of being able to do so

- Gain a deeper understanding about your body

- Achieve your target weight

- Free yourself from the hassle of food preparation

Know exactly what your objectives are before starting IF as it will also help you create a plan that will lead you to your preferred results. However, you also have to take note that no matter how good your goals are, you can't expect intermittent fasting to work effectively and safely in achieving them if you are also doing the following:

- **Using "health" as an excuse for your eating disorder or for strictly controlling your food intake**
- **Fasting too often for extremely long periods of time**

- Exercising excessively or having insufficient sleep

- Over-obsessing with food or binging once your feeding or eating period arrives

- Taking appetite suppressants to avoid extreme difficulty during the fasting period

- Using intermittent fasting as an excuse for overeating or unhealthy and poor food choices and eating patterns

You have to set healthy goals for adapting intermittent fasting. Avoid doing it to compromise your health. The first thing to do is to set a healthy goal than learn the basics of nutrition. Make sure to consume healthy and high-quality foods at the right time and amounts.

Choose the right foods

During your eating period, it is important to eat the right foods. Make each calorie that your body takes in count. In case you choose an IF pattern, which gives you the chance to take in calories during the fasting state, then go for nutrient-dense foods, particularly those with high amounts of healthy fats, fiber, and protein. Some examples are eggs, avocado, nuts, fish, beans, and lentils.

You should also pick nutrient-dense foods rich in fiber, minerals, vitamins, and other essential nutrients that can stabilize your blood sugar during the eating period. The foods should help prevent nutritional deficiency. It is also advisable to pick filling foods with low calorie content, like raw vegetables and popcorn. You can also include fruits that have high water content, like melon and grapes in your meals.

To enjoy the fed state, make sure to improve the taste of the foods you are planning to eat without necessarily increasing their calorie content. You can do that by generously seasoning your meals with herbs, vinegar, spices, and garlic. This will allow your foods to be filled with flavor without increasing calories. It also helps in reducing your hunger.

Ensure that you stay hydrated, too. Drink enough water and low-calorie drinks, like herbal teas all throughout the day.

Do not pressure yourself to perfect the eating pattern

Avoid freaking out and pressuring yourself to perfect everything, especially if you are still a beginner in IF. If you intend to follow the 16/8 rule, for instance, then do not freak out in case you were just able to fast for 14 to 15 hours on a particular day. Do not also bombard yourself with unnecessary questions, like whether or not the result will be ruined in case you ate one apple during your fasting period.

To make the whole eating pattern more manageable, try to relax. Keep in mind that the human body is a machinery that learns to adapt as time goes by. You cannot expect it to follow the routine right away, especially if you are still new to it. Do not force yourself to stick to really rigid fasting rules. For instance, if you wish to enjoy eating your breakfast one day and fast on another, then allow yourself to do it.

Note that while you need to be more disciplined, especially if you really want to lose weight, you should avoid freaking out and worrying and stressing over every minute detail of the process. Just relax and you will notice your body starting to adapt to the new routine and the IF working in your favor slowly but surely.

Listen to your body

If you intend to stick to intermittent fasting for quite a long period then make it a point to listen and observe the cues sent to you by your body. Some of the cues you have to watch out for are significant changes in your satiety, hunger, and appetite, such as food cravings, your emotional or mental health and mood, the quality of your sleep, your athletic performance, and your energy levels. Make it a point to observe your immunity, hormonal health, blood profile, and the way you look, too.

Observing and listening to your body can help you figure out whether IF is working for you. If you are into strength training, then you have to listen to body cues even more. Find out if you experience lightheadedness during your workout. If that happens, it would be helpful to consume enough water.

Also, act right away if there is a noticeable drop in your performance. If that is the case, make it a point to consume enough calories, particularly those coming from protein and healthy fats during your eating window. Stop working out if your body feels extremely off. Allow yourself to have time to ease and get used to fasted workouts and IF. This tip is even more important, especially for endurance athletes.

Avoid overdoing your workouts

Just like what we have talked about in the previous tips, it is necessary to listen to the signals sent by your body. This is all the more necessary if you decide to combine your workout with fasting. Note that intermittent fasting and regular workout combined can produce better and quicker weight loss results. However, you should avoid overdoing your workouts, so you will not end up harming your body.

If you wish to work out and pair it with IF, then make sure to take into consideration all the things that are happening in your life. Consider the specific amount and intensity of training and exercise you do. Consider your rest and recovery period, too. You should also take into consideration the suitability of intermittent fasting with your normal social activities and regular routines as well as the other stress and demands that life throws at you. By considering all these factors, you can figure out what type of workout is compatible with your lifestyle and your preferred IF method.

Do not deprive yourself

Your decision to practice intermittent fasting does not necessarily mean that you should deprive yourself with even a drink during your fasted period. Note that it is okay to drink water and zero-calorie beverages. You can drink black coffee, tea, or water when you are fasting. Do not also stop yourself from putting something in your drink (like milk in your coffee).

Furthermore, remember that you are also allowed to drink diet soda on an occasional basis when you are fasting. Note that the goal here is habit-building and consistency. This means that if you feel like you can go through the fasting period more easily with a cream or milk in your coffee then there is no reason to deprive yourself.

Also, remember that adhering to the routine 80 percent of the time for a whole year is actually better than adhering to it 100 percent but only abandoning it after just a few weeks due to it being too rigid and restrictive. You can be stricter if you intend to reach a minimum percentage of body fat. However, if you want to achieve your goal at your own pace then do the things that you think will make you remain compliant to it for a long time.

Eat filling and satiating meals

Your meals can greatly affect your ability to stick to your fasting and dieting routines. This is the main reason why you have to make sure that the meals and foods you eat during the eating window are all filling and satiating. Among the foods that can satisfy and fill you up during your eating window are eggs, yogurt, potatoes, oatmeal, bananas and soups.

You may also eat those foods that you can consume in large amounts without taking in a lot of calories, including legumes, fruits and veggies. This does not mean, however, that you should go all out when it comes to eating. You should still try limiting yourself without over-deprivation. This will allow you to enjoy your experience when following your chosen intermittent fasting method, thereby allowing you to stick to it for quite a long period.

Keep yourself busy

Your boredom will be your number one enemy when you are doing intermittent fasting that's why you have to do something to keep yourself busy during your fasting period. Boredom is also the silent killer, which might destroy your progress gradually. It might cause you to eat more than what is recommended without even realising it. It is mainly because of dopamine, one of the chemicals in your brain, which can make you feel good each time you accomplish something.

This chemical is also responsible for the behaviour motivated by reward.

It has been discovered that eating is actually a major factor in encouraging your body to release dopamine, producing the positive feelings as a result. In most cases, unhealthy and junk foods, especially those rich in sodium, fat, and sugar, are the ones that can make you feel great. Therefore, if you are bored during your fasting period then there is a great possibility that you will grab a food no matter how hard you resist the temptation.

With that in mind, make sure that you are busy with something during the fasting period. Do not just sit around and think about your hunger since you may only struggle in the end. It would also be best to time your fasting period in a way that you can maximise its efficiency and minimise discomfort. For instance, schedule it after you have eaten a nice dinner so you have more time to fast without having to think about food since it is already close to your bedtime.

Develop an exit strategy

If you wish to follow intermittent fasting for a long time, then make sure to develop a plan that will guide and help you in reintroducing a regular eating schedule into your daily routines. Avoid committing the mistakes of those who fasted in the past who tend to trip up after deciding to break free from the IF cycle since they have a hard time reacquainting with their own hunger signals and appetite.

With that in mind, it would be a big help to develop an exit plan once you are done with intermittent fasting, especially if you prefer to do it the mindful and healthy way. You should also keep track of your progress and the results of practicing IF, too, so you will know exactly when the right time to stop is.

Intermittent fasting is indeed an incredible eating pattern, especially for those who wish to lose weight. The problem is that while others can easily do the fast without trouble and without experiencing too many irresistible food temptations, there are also those who find the whole process difficult. If you feel like you need a bit of help to succeed then you can always apply the tips mentioned in this chapter.

That way, you have a better chance of keeping your hunger at bay, preventing mindless eating even if you are hungry, gaining full control of your nutrition, and sticking to the routine, thereby allowing you to enjoy and maximise its results.

Intermittent Fasting Myths

Intermittent fasting is one of the most rewarding eating patterns and lifestyle you can try. However, before starting your journey towards enjoying its numerous benefits, it is crucial to study the facts and myths behind it. This chapter will debunk some of the most famous intermittent fasting myths and offer truthful information about how this eating pattern really works.

Myth #1 – Intermittent fasting guarantees significant weight loss.

Contrary to what most people believe, IF can't be expected to result in significant weight loss all the time. This is especially true if you are doing this approach the wrong way. Note that regardless of the length of your fast, you can't still expect to achieve the results you want as far as weight loss is concerned if you constantly include burgers, candies, pizzas, and other unhealthy foods during your eating period. You still need to pair IF with regular exercises and a healthy diet. You can't treat each eating period as a cheat day.

Myth #2 – Intermittent fasting leads to muscle loss.

No, your muscles will not shrivel up and break down during your fasted state. Keep in mind that the human body stores two forms of energy, namely fat and sugar. This means that your body will only be using these two forms of stored energy.

Protein, which is a major component of your muscles, will not be used by your body to produce energy when you are fasting. What happens, instead, is that your body will make use of sugar as the primary source of fuel during the first 1-2 days without food.

After that, your body will begin opening up and accessing stored fats as a source of energy. This means that it will start breaking down the stored fats in your body to create fuel once your stored sugar depletes. Each person has around 50,000 to 100,000 calorics of fat on average stored in his body, which is equal to almost one month's worth of available stored fats.

If you intend to fast, therefore, then you do not have to worry about your muscles breaking down since it is your stored fat and sugar that your body will use as fuel.

Myth #3 – Intermittent fasting can slow down your metabolism.

You do not have to worry about intermittent fasting negatively affecting your metabolic rate. It is because the entire eating pattern will not slow down your metabolism. Keep in mind that IF does not involve excessive calorie restrictions. What it does is to restrict the time you consume calories.

A few more hours spent waiting to take your first meal does not have a major effect on your metabolic rate. However, you should avoid under-eating during your eating period as this practice is the one that might send your metabolism downhill.

Myth #4 – Intermittent fasting can lead to poor brain performance.

Glucose is your brain's main source of fuel. With that in mind, it is no longer surprising to see those who are planning to try IF worrying about being unable to give their brain a consistent supply of glucose. The truth, however, is that IF will not negatively affect the performance of your brain.

Keep in mind that your body is still capable of using stored fuel from your body to produce glucose. This means that even if you follow low-carb intermittent fasting approach, it is still possible for your brain to get a good supply of fuel through ketone bodies that break down fat.

Intermittent fasting can even lead to better mental performance, focus, and clarity. It is mainly because fasting can stimulate epinephrine and norepinephrine production. If you get into the fasting mode, your body will cause a minor stress response, which releases adrenaline. This breaks down the fats stored in your body as fuel, thereby providing you with the focus and energy you need.

Furthermore, fasting can lead to the production of BDNF (brain-derived neurotropic factor). This can help your existing neurons survive, stimulate the growth of new neurons, and improve your learning and thinking ability and your memory. It also helps lessen your risk of suffering from depression and Alzheimer's disease.

Myth #5 – You have limitless options during your eating window.

Some of those who tried intermittent fasting wrongly believed that they are allowed to eat whatever they want provided they consume it during the eating window. This is actually not true. In fact, eating without limitations during the eating window can only have serious consequences to your health, wellness, and weight loss goals. Eating anything during the eating period might cause your body to get confused.

It is because from being on a fasting state that results in balanced levels of blood glucose and fat burning, your body suddenly experiences a spike in insulin and blood glucose. If this happens, you are just basically ruining the incredible effort you have exerted for fasting.

Furthermore, not controlling the amount of food you eat during your eating window can make you feel terrible and produce issues, like weight gain, mood swings, and hormonal imbalance. Note that while intermittent fasting does not require you to be extremely strict during your eating window, you still have to balance the foods you eat. It is still crucial to apply moderation as this can help you gather the results you want from IF.

Myth #6 – Intermittent fasting is the sole reason for macronutrient deficiency.

Remember that if you follow your preferred intermittent fasting method the right way, you do not have to worry about experiencing nutrient deficiency. In fact, fasting is not the main reason for nutrient deficiency. Diet plans that are deficient in nutrients are actually the culprit. You will not suffer from nutrient deficiency if you actually stick to eating whole, balanced, and nutritious foods during your eating window.

You do not have to worry too much about your body not getting enough nutrients when you are fasting as there is no basis for such claim. In fact, fasting can cause your body to create nutrient efficiency. It increases the possibility of your body utilizing less nutrients, thereby retaining them so your body can efficiently use them in the future.

With that in mind, fasting can't be pointed as the culprit for nutrient deficiency but poor diet, chronic stress, unstable blood sugar levels, leaky gut syndrome, and low levels of stomach acid.

Myth #7 – Intermittent fasting can lead to overeating.

This is not true. What actually dictates your unhealthy eating behaviour includes leptin and blood sugar. Having unstable blood sugar levels can cause food cravings, especially if your sugar crashes down. Being desensitised to leptin can also result in difficulties figuring out whether you have already consumed enough foods.

Leptin actually refers to a signalling hormone within your body, which plays a huge role in controlling your hunger. Certain factors, like chronic calorie restriction, poor quality of sleep, binge eating, and stress can lead to leptin resistance, causing you to be at a higher risk of overeating.

Instead of causing you to overeat, intermittent fasting can actually stabilise your blood sugar and improve your sensitivity to leptin. This can further improve your ability to control overeating or binge eating.

Myth #8 – You won't be able to exercise if you are fasting.

This is a misconception since it is actually safe for you to exercise even if you are on your fasting period. Working out will not result in muscle wasting or loss. In fact, fasted workouts can lead to the growth of your muscles provided you still consume adequate amounts of protein and calories every day.

In addition, working out while fasting can also produce other incredible benefits, including improved ketosis state, better fat burning ability, and increased growth hormone levels. Just make sure to stay hydrated if you intend to do some high-intensity exercises during your fasting state. In case you wish to gain muscles, then it would be helpful to take essential amino acid supplements.

Myth #9 – Intermittent fasting can lead to starving and irritability.

A lot of those who haven't tried intermittent fasting yet but want to do it for health reasons are often concerned about getting irritable if they experience extreme hunger. While this statement bears some weight, note that it is only true on a temporary basis.

You may experience irritability and hunger at first, especially if you are used to eating at least three meals spaced periodically every day. This may happen because you are still adjusting to your new eating routine/pattern.

You can't expect this to happen permanently, though. You can slowly make the adjustments by doing simple fasting routines or by doing it for one to two times every week at first. This will allow you to introduce the routine to your system. You can then slowly increase the number and duration of your fasting sessions as soon as you feel comfortable.

You do not have to rush things. Allow your body to adapt so you will not end up experiencing too much hunger and irritability. Once you are fully adjusted with this eating pattern, you can start enjoying its numerous benefits like better mental clarity and mood.

Myth #10 – Intermittent fasting does not work for those suffering from diabetes.

Another myth associated with fasting that you have to be aware of is that it is ineffective for diabetics. It is because most people are made to believe that they need to consume foods constantly as a means of maintaining their blood sugar level. The truth, however, is that IF works for those suffering from Type 2 diabetes, especially in improving weight loss results and stabilising blood sugar.

There is even a possibility for prolonged fasting to restore their sensitivity to insulin. You may also combine IF with a ketogenic diet if you want to further improve its ability to restore your sensitivity to insulin. What is good about having improved insulin sensitivity is that your body will no longer need to produce too much insulin. This results in minimal inflammation, which is a big help for diabetics and those who are prone to developing kidney and heart diseases.

Type 1 diabetes sufferers who are incapable of producing insulin, however, should closely keep track of their blood sugar level before practicing intermittent fasting so they can do it correctly. They can still fast for around 12-16 hours every day but this will depend on the stability of their blood sugar level.

Motivation for you While Intermittent Fasting

It is understood that it is not always easy to stay on a diet. Although the intermittent fast cannot be thought of as a diet, it requires you to make lifestyle and food choices that can be a little taxing at times.

In this chapter, we will look at simple things that you can do to stick with the fast.

Expectations

It is obvious that you will have a lot of expectations from the diet. It is normal to have them, as you will want to reach your ideal weight within a certain period of time. But what is important to note is that you have to have realistic expectations when it comes to the time frame you set to achieve the weight loss. You cannot achieve it overnight. If you are obese now, then try to go for a 6 to 12-month plan to lose weight. If you go for something lesser then it might not work out for you. If you set an unrealistic goal and see that it is not working out for you then you will feel discouraged and might want to go off the diet. It is therefore important to set realistic goals in order to achieve them better.

Motivators

Make sure you know exactly why you are going for the weight loss routine. It is obvious that you will want to lose weight and fit into smaller clothes etc. But apart from these, there have to be other motivators as well that will keep you on track. Make a list of them and stick them in your room or have a copy of the list on your phone so that you can look at it and remain motivated. These will keep you from going for something unhealthy and sticking with the fast.

Clear out the kitchen

A top tip is to get rid of all junk and processed foods from the kitchen. These can be quite tempting. Follow the rule, "out of sight, out of mind." Go through everything in the kitchen and get rid of all items that are bad for the diet. Keep it off the shelves and off the counters. Replace them with healthier alternatives such as nuts. Make sure you do not go into the kitchen after a certain point in time say 10 or 11 at night. Once you have had your last meal, stay away from the kitchen area. If you have a lot of junk and processed food lying around then throw a party to finish it all in one go.

Don't be too harsh

Don't be too harsh on yourself if you end up going for a cheat meal. It can be a little difficult to make a sudden change in your lifestyle. It is therefore advisable to go slow with it. Make sure you ease into the diet so that you can stave off temptations. Do not be tempted to fall off the wagon just because you had one cheat meal. Treat it as a cheat and focus on your fast.

Carry your food

Do not forget to carry your meals everywhere you go. Be it to the office or to a party, you have to carry the meals with you so that you can avoid the hassle of settling for something that is forbidden by the diet. If you don't have a ready snack with you then you are bound to go for something unhealthy. Have a high-protein snack ready that you can bite into as soon as you get hungry. A few good options include peanuts, almonds and a hard-boiled egg. These can keep you going until the next meal.

Don't go for too much

If you are just starting out with the fast then make sure you go slowly. Do not do too many things at once, as that will confuse your body. If you do not exercise at all then go for simple ones at first. Once you have settled into the diet, go for an exercise routine. If you start both at once then you will do justice to neither. But make sure at some point you take up exercising and do not rely on the fast alone. It would be best to wait for about a month before taking up an exercise regime. Although research suggests you have to stick to something for at least a month for the habit to stick, it is best you take it up seriously and continue for at least 6 months to a year.

Do your research

It is obvious that in this day and age nobody can go without eating out. It can be quite a challenge to go out and not find something edible on the menu. In such a case, it pays to do your research and make sure you find a restaurant that serves meals that cater to your choice. It will be even better if you find something that customises the menu for you. If you are traveling, then plan ahead and find out which places you can eat at. Pack enough food to keep you going for at least 3 days. Make sure you go for foods that can last at least a week.

Reward yourself

It is always important to reward yourself with something nice for keeping up the good work. It can be a trip to the spa or a vacation. You can also buy yourself something that you have always wanted like a crock-pot or an air fryer. A recipe book too can serve as a reward. The reward can be anything as long as you feel motivated to keep up with the diet. It would be advisable not to go for a cheat meal as a reward.

Mindfulness and meditation

Mindfulness is a technique that helps you dig deep into your thoughts and remain completely focused on the task at hand. By practicing mindful eating, you give yourself the chance to enjoy a healthy meal. Those who enjoy their meals are able to better connect with the food and lose a significant amount of weight just by remaining focused on the meal. Another research found that mindfulness successfully put an end to binge eating. It is said to have reduced from almost 4 to 1.5 times a week over a period of 6 weeks. It is, therefore, a good idea to indulge in mindfulness eating. You can also engage in meditation. This can keep your mind calm. Try to stay away from stress as much as possible as it can negatively impact your health. It can also cause you to gain weight. The more stress free you remain, the better off you are in terms of attaining weight loss.

Keep track

Keep track of your progress. This can serve as a big motivator to keep you on track. Maintain a diary and write down everything including your weight, measurements, meal timings, meal plans, etc. Refer back to it from time to time to ensure that you are on the right track. It is a good idea to maintain a blog and keep updating your progress. Your friends and family members can access it and encourage you to keep up the good work.

Partner up

Getting a partner is always a great way to remain motivated to stick to a fast. Not only will you have company, you will also remain motivated to keep t it. It can be a spouse, partner, sibling, colleague, friend, etc., as long as they wish to benefit from the fast. Usually, when one partner decides to make a healthy choice be it dietary modification or exercise, the other decides to follow as well. You will also find it easier with your partner chipping in to prepare the healthy meals and keeping track of your progress.

Go for a heavy breakfast

There is nothing better than a healthy and hearty breakfast or rather the first meal of the day. If you plan on having your meal by 12 noon then go for something that is loaded with proteins and other nutrients. As per studies, women who ate 1.05 ounces of protein for breakfast were able to avoid feeling peckish before lunch as compared to those who ate a breakfast low in proteins. You can also have a protein and fiber rich lunch to supplement the breakfast.

Take your time

Don't be in a hurry to get through everything at once. Go about it in a slow and steady manner. As mentioned earlier, it might take at least a month for you to make a habit stick. Be patient with it. Keep at it for at least 6 months. Do not compare yourself to others. If there are people passing negative comments, then learn to ignore them. You have to remain focused and motivated to achieve the slimmer, fitter and better you.

Customize

Customise the diet for yourself. Only you will know your body best. Do not follow what someone else is following as what works for them might not work for you. It is best to come up with a plan that is sustainable in the long run as compared to one that will only provide you momentary results.

These are just some of the things you can do to remain motivated. Do not limit it to just these and do whatever it takes for you to stick with the intermittent fast.

CHAPTER 8: 16 BEST METHODS TO GET THE MOST OUT OF THIS DIET

Before you can start practicing Intermittent Fasting and incorporating it into your lifestyle, you'll have to know all the possibilities so you can choose the right one(s) for yourself, your goals, your habits, and your body/personality type. Read through the following 10 suggestions to find which methods sound most right to you.

Lean-Gains Method

The lean-gains method essentially focuses on the combined efforts of rigorous exercise, fasting, and a healthy diet. The fame surrounding this approach comes from its acclaimed success at turning fat directly into muscle. The goal is to fast within each day for 14-16 hours, starting when you wake up.

The ideal approach to lean-gains seems to be that you wake up and fast until 1 pm, doing some stretches and pre-workout warmups just before noon. Starting at noon, you would engage in training in whatever exercise you choose for an hour or less, ending with you breaking fast around 1 pm. Your meal at this time would be the largest of the day.

You would engage in your day as normal past then, as possible, eating again around 4 pm, then eating for the final time around 9 pm, giving yourself a ~15-hour fast until the next day at 1 pm. If you choose this approach yet feel a bit overwhelmed, you can work up to 15 hours, starting with a 13- or 14-hour fast only for the first week, building up to 15- or 16-hour fasting after that.

16:8 method is one of the most popular methods among Intermittent Fasters. Essentially, you spend 16 hours within each day fasting, and the other 8 hours are your eating window. Most people try to choose their 8-hour eating window to be the times when they're primarily active. If you're a night person, feel free to make it a little later. Hold off eating during the daytime as much as possible then breakfast around 3 or 4 pm. For morning people, breakfast earlier, say, around 11 am, stopping food consumption by 7 pm.

16:8 is an incredibly flexible method that works for many different kinds of people. It's even flexible once you decide to try a particular fasting to eating window ratio. For example, if you don't seem to be jiving with the 11-7pm eating window, you can absolutely alter the next day to suit your needs better. Maybe try waiting until later in the day to breakfast! Try what you need to do, as long as you're keeping to that 16:8-hour ratio.

Whereas lean-gains method technically applies the same hourly ratio, it's much more strict regarding healthy diet and exercise regimen. 16:8 method does not need any type of exercise booster, but that's up to the practitioner. It is always best to try adding healthy dietary choices to one's IF eating schedule but don't try to restrict too many calories, as it can incorporate to feelings of lightheadedness and low energy. With 16:8, you can eat what you need and swap the hours around as desired.

14:10 Method

Similar to 16:8 method, 14:10 requires fasting and eating in varying degrees within each day. In this case, you would fast for 14 hours and engage in eating for a 10-hour window afterward. This method has the same flexibility as 16:8 in terms of what time of day it's arranged around, and how easy it is to troubleshoot. But it's additionally flexible in the sense that the eating window is two hours longer, accommodating people with more intense physical routines or daily demands, as well as people who simply need to eat a little later in the day to feel well.

20:4 Method

Whereas 14:10 method was an easier step **down** from 16:8 method, 20:4 method is definitely a step **up** in terms of difficulty. It's a more intense method certainly, for it requires 20 hours of fasting within each day with only a 4-hour eating window for the individual to gain all his or her nutrients and energy.

Most people who try this method end up having either one large meal with several snacks or they have two smaller meals with fewer snacks. 20:4 is flexible in that sense—the sense whereby the individual chooses how the eating window is divided amongst meals and snacks.

20:4 method is tricky, for many people instinctually over-eat during the eating window, but that's neither necessary nor is it healthy. People that choose 20:4 method should try to keep meal portions around the same size that they would normally have been without fasting. Experimenting on how many snacks are needed will be helpful as well with this method.

Many people end up working up to 20:4 from other methods, based on what their bodies can handle and what they're ready to attempt. Few start with 20:4, so if it's not working for you right away, please don't be too hard on yourself! Step it back to 16:8 and then see how soon you can get back to where you'd like to be.

The warrior method is quite similar to 20:4 method in that the individual fasts for 20 hours within each day and breaks fast for a 4-hour eating window. The difference is in the outlook and mindset of the practitioner, however. Essentially, the thought process behind warrior method is that, in ancient times, the hunter coming home from stalking prey or the warrior coming home from battle would really only get one meal each day. One meal would have to provide sustenance for the rest of the day, recuperative energy from the ordeal, and sustainable energy for the future.

Therefore, practitioners of warrior method are encouraged to have one large meal when they breakfast, and that meal should be jam-packed with fats, proteins, and carbs for the rest of the day (and for the days ahead). Just like with 20:4 method, however, it can sometimes be too intense for practitioners, and it's very easy to scale this one back in forcefulness by making up a method like 18:6 or 17:7. If it's not working, don't force it to work past two weeks, but do try to make it through a week to see if it's your stubbornness or if it's just a mismatch with the method.

12:12 Method

12:12 method is a little easier, along with the lines of 14:10, rather than 16:8 or 20:4. Beginners to Intermittent Fasting would do well to try this one right off the bat. Some people get 12 hours of sleep each night and can easily wake up from the fasting period, ready to engage with the eating window. Many people use this method in their lives without even knowing it.

To go about 12:12 method in your life, however, you'll want to be as purposeful about it as you can be. Make sure to be strict about your 12-hour cut-offs. Make sure it's working and feeling good in your body, and then you're invited to take things up a notch and try, say, 14:10 or maybe your own invention, like 15:11. As always, start with what works and then move up (or down) to what feels right (and even possibly **better**).

5:2 Method

5:2 method is popular among those who want to take things up a notch generally. Instead of fasting and eating within each day, these individuals take up a practice of fasting two whole days out of the week. The other 5 days are free to eat, exercise, or diet as desired, but those other two days (which can be consecutive or scattered throughout the week) must be strictly fasting days.

For those fasting days, it's not as if the individual can't eat anything altogether, however. In actuality, one is allowed to consume no more than 500 calories each day for this Intermittent Fasting method. I suppose these fasting days would be better referred to as "restricted-intake" days, for that is a more accurate description.

5:2 method is extremely rewarding, but it is also one of the more difficult ones to attempt. If you're having issues with this method, don't be afraid to experiment the next week with a method like 14:10 or 16:8, where you're fasting and eating within each day. If that works better for you, don't be ashamed to embrace it! However, if you're dedicated to having days "on" and days "off" with fasting and eating, there are other alternatives, too.

Eat-Stop-Eat (24-Hour) Method

The eat-stop-eat or 24-hour method is another option for people who want to have days "on" and "off" between fasting and eating. It's a little less intense than 5:2 method, and it's much more flexible for the individual, based on what he or she needs. For instance, if you need a literal 24-hour fast each week and that's it, you can do that. On the other hand, if you want a more flexible 5:2 method-type thing to happen, you can work with what you want and create a method surrounding those desires and goals.

The most successful approaches to the eat-stop-eat method have involved more strict dieting (or at the very least, cautious and healthy eating) during the 5 or 6 days when the individual engages in the week's free-eating window. For the individual to truly see success with weight loss, there will have to be some caloric restriction (or high nutrition focus) those 5 or 6 days, too, so that the body will have a version of consistency in health and nutrition content.

On the one or two days each week the individual decides to fast, there can still be highly-restricted caloric intake. As with 5:2 method, he or she can consume no more than 500 calories worth of food and drink during these fasting days so that the body can maintain energy flow and more.

If the individual engages in exercise, those workout days should absolutely be reserved for the 5 or 6 free-eating days. The same goes for 5:2 method. Try not to exercise (at least not excessively) on those days that are chosen for fasting. Your body will not appreciate the added stress when you're taking in so few calories. As always, you can choose to move up from eat-stop-eat to another method if this works easily and you're interested in something more. Furthermore, you can start with a strict 24-hour method and then move up to a more flexible eat-stop-eat approach! Do what feels right, and never be afraid to troubleshoot one method for the sake of choosing another.

Alternate-Day Method

The alternate-day method is similar to eat-stop-eat and 5:2 methods because it focuses on individual days "on" and "off" for fasting and eating. The difference for this method, in particular, is that it ends up being at least 2 days a week fasting, and sometimes, it can be as many as 4.

Some people follow very strict approaches to alternate-day method and literally fast every other day, only consuming 500 calories or less on those days designated for fasting. Some people, on the other hand, are much more flexible, and they tend to go for two days eating, one day fasting, two days eating, one day fasting, etc. The alternate-day method is even more flexible than eat-stop-eat in that sense, for it allows the individual to choose how he or she alternates between eating and fasting, based on what works for the body and mind the best.

The alternate-day method is like a step up from eat-stop-eat and 24-hour methods, especially if the individual truly alternates one-day fasting and the next day eating, etc. This more intense style of fasting works particularly well for people who are working on equally intense fitness regimens, surprisingly. People who are eating more calories a day than 2000 (which is true for a lot of bodybuilders and fitness buffs) will have more to gain from the alternate-day method, for you only have to cut back your eating on fasting days to about 25% of your standard caloric intake. Therefore, those fasting days can still provide solid nutritional support for fitness experts while helping them sculpt their bodies and maintain a new level of health.

Spontaneous Skipping Method

Alternate-day method and eat-stop-eat method are certainly flexible in their approaches to when the individual fasts and when he or she eats. However, none of those mentioned above plans are quite as flexible as spontaneous skipping method. Spontaneous skipping method literally only requires that the individual skip meals within each day, whenever desired (and when it's sensed that the body can handle it).

Many people with more sensitive digestive systems or who practice more intense fitness regimens will start their experiences with IF through spontaneous skipping method before moving on to something more intensive. People who have very haphazard daily schedules or people who are around food a lot but forget to eat will benefit from this method, for it works well with chaotic schedules and unplanned energies.

Despite that chaotic and unorganised potential, spontaneous skipping method can also be more structured and organised, depending on what you make of it! For instance, someone desiring more structure can choose which meal each day they'd like to skip. Let's say he chooses to skip breakfast each day. Then, his spontaneous skipping method will be structured around making sure to skip breakfast (a.k.a.—not to eat until at least 12 pm) daily. Whatever you need to do to make this method work, try it! This method is made for experimentation and adventurousness.

Crescendo Method

The final method worth mentioning is crescendo method, which is very well-suited for female practitioners (since their anatomies can be so detrimentally sensitive to high-intensity fasts). Essentially, this approach is made for internal awareness, gentle introductions, and gradual additions, depending on what works and what doesn't. It's a very active, trial-and-error type of method.

Through crescendo method, the individual starts by only fasting 2 or 3 days a week, and on those fast days, it wouldn't be a very intense fast at all. In fact, it wouldn't even be so strict that the individual would have to consume no more than 500 calories, like with 5:2, eat-stop-eat, and others. Instead, these "fasting" days would be trial periods for methods like 12:12, 14:10, 16:8, or 20:4. The remaining 4 or 5 days out of the week would be open eating-window periods, but again, the practitioner is encouraged to maintain a healthy diet throughout the week.

Crescendo method works extremely well for female practitioners because it enables them to see how methods like 14:10 or 12:12 will affect their bodies without tying them to the method hook, line, and sinker. It allows them to see what each method does to their hormone levels, their menstruation tendencies, and their mood swings. Therefore, the crescendo method encourages these people to be more in touch with their bodies before moving too quickly into something that could do serious anatomical and hormonal damage.

Crescendo method will work extremely well for overweight or diabetic practitioners, too, for it will allow them to have these same "trial period" moments with all the methods before choosing what feels and works best, based on each individual situation.

Making Your Choice

When you make your choice from the 10 different options listed above, there are several things you'll want to keep in mind. First and foremost, amongst those things will be the fact that you can always choose another method (or a more flexible one to start with) in case something doesn't work as you'd hoped. You can **always** troubleshoot your method in this way, and there's more on this topic in chapter 9 for those interested in troubleshooting (as well as for those being forced by their bodies to troubleshoot ASAP).

Ultimately, you'll also want to keep the following points in mind as you go about selecting your method: body type & abilities, lifestyle, daily tendencies, work routine, friends & family, and dietary choices.

For all these considerations, remember what feels best to you, and remember to keep your goals with IF in mind at all times! If you ever feel like you're sacrificing your sanity or bodily health to attain these goals, go back to that step of troubleshooting, for you should never need to sacrifice those things to achieve any type of goals. Essentially, keep your eye on the prize and remember to choose what feels right and see what works from there.

Consider your body type and abilities. Think of how your body looks and feels and how much about it you'd like to change. Think about how you react to food and what it looks like when you're hungry. Think about those things you view as your "limits" and how comfortable you are with pushing. Are you a fitness freak or a couch potato? Are you huskier or slimmer? Does your body hold onto fat or build muscle quickly? Do you retain water weight or not? Do you work out? Do you require a lot of water when you do? Consider all these things about your body and more, then compare them to the methods listed above. Compare them, too, to your overall goals with Intermittent Fasting to make sure that you're choosing a method that will help you actualise those goals as you conceive of them. If you're looking to lose weight quickly, try a method that works with days "on" and "off" between fasting and eating. If you're looking to build muscle, lean-gains method is probably the choice for you! If you're looking to boost your brain and heart, start with crescendo method and see where it takes you!

Consider your lifestyle. When do you normally wake up and how much sleep do you get on an average night? How hungry are you normally when you do wake up? How fast is your metabolism and when do you notice its peak? How do you make your living? Do you spend a lot of time in the car or on your feet or in an office? Are you constantly around other people or are you often alone? When you choose your method for Intermittent Fasting, make sure to consider all these lifestyle points. Maybe you wouldn't want to choose to time with a method that disallows you to eat when you normally need the most energy. Maybe you wouldn't want to choose a method that forces you to eat when you're supposed to be at work. Most of these methods have a degree of choice and flexibility, so when you do find one you like, remember that you don't have to put yourself in positions that go against your nature (or circadian rhythms) to achieve any of your goals. Stay flexible, keep your goals in mind, and respect the norms of your body!

Consider your daily tendencies. Do you eat mostly in the daylight hours or after the sun goes down? Do you go to work in the daytime or nighttime? Are you generally nocturnal, diurnal, or crepuscular? Do you have a lot of freedom and flexibility in your daily routines? Do you travel a lot for work? Do you spend a lot of time on the move? Do you have trouble remembering to eat? Are you the type of person that works out on the regular? Consider these themes in your life and more before you choose your method. Does it make sense for you to have low intake days where you consume 500 calories or less? Or does it make more sense for you to have extended periods in each day where you're just not eating based on your habits or tendencies or otherwise? Plan something that makes sense and respects your habits so that the transition into Intermittent Fasting is as easy and painless as possible.

Consider your work routine. Do you go to work in the morning or night? Are you allowed to eat at work? Do you work around food or in the food service industry? Do you work on your feet all day or by doing something strenuous? Do you receive purposeful or accidental exercise opportunities at work or are you just sitting in the same position all day? All these elements of your work routine will be important to consider as you decide which avenue of Intermittent Fasting to go down. You won't want to engage in a method like 20:4 if you're at work every day for incredibly short shifts. 20:4 works better for someone who works very long and distracting days. You won't want to try a method like 12:12 if part of your eating window involves being at work, when you're not allowed to eat at work. Remember to take your work life, routines, and restrictions into account when you go about making this choice, for you will make things much less harsh on yourself if you can look at this bigger picture from the beginning and planning stages.

Consider your friends, coworkers, and family. How loud are their opinions? Are their lives oriented toward health? Do they demean you a lot or make fun of your choices? Or are they encouraging all the time? Are these people your support system or are they your devils' advocates? Do you have the sense that they want to see you succeed? On the most basic level, are they nice to you and respectful of your choices? It might not seem that important, but the attitudes and supportive capacity of your friends, coworkers, and family can mean **the world** when you make a big choice like starting Intermittent Fasting in your life. Sometimes, people just don't want to see us succeed. They block our successes with jealousy, pride, ignorance, or arrogance. When friends and family act like this, it's better to choose a method that allows you to avoid discussing IF around them whatsoever. When friends and family are open and supportive, they shouldn't influence your choice that much at all; it's just when things are tenuous that you'll need to keep them (and your time around them) in consideration.

Finally, **consider your dietary choices**. Do you eat a lot of processed foods? Or do you eat a largely whole-foods, plant-based diet? Do you count calories? Do you cautiously skim nutrition facts? Are you looking for something specific like high fat, high fiber, or high protein? Are you hoping to change your diet entirely or are you trying to keep things the way they are? Are you willing to sacrifice items of your diet to actualise your goals? All these questions help determine which type of method you're going to be ready for. Essentially, if you're trying to change your diet entirely, a method with days "on" and days "off" will work best for you. In this case, try 5:2, alternate-day, eat-stop-eat, and spontaneous skip methods. However, if you don't want to change your diet that much at all, a method where you fast for periods within each day will be desirable instead. Try methods like 20:4, 16:8, 14:10, or 12:12 for this type of situation.

As long as you make your selection with these 6 points in mind, you're sure to succeed with your Intermittent Fasting goals. You enable yourself to make the safest, smartest, best choice for your circumstances, and that's an incredible tool to use in so many different applications. In this case, it's a tool that will help keep you healthy, boost your brain, heal your heart, and shed that excess weight like melted butter!

As a reminder, your first choice still might not be the absolute **right one**, but by making the most educated choice possible, you're sure to start from a good place and learn a lot about yourself regardless. Make sure you have a runner-up method (or two!) that's easy to swap to just in case the first one doesn't seem to show progress. Work smarter, not harder! Plan ahead, do the research and know yourself. These are the truest steps to success that I know. And as always, don't be afraid to check with your doctor or nutritionist once the choice has been made. They'll be able to give you the final affirmation you need so you can get started on your new, healthy lifestyle with Intermittent Fasting in no time!

CHAPTER 9: HOW TO TRACK YOUR DIET USING VARIOUS FREE APPLICATIONS

Things can become confusing, especially at first, when you start with intermittent fasting. This is why using some essential tools to help you keep track of everything would be a good idea. You can always go old school and decide to plot down your schedule on a piece of paper. Perhaps buy a new notebook that is dedicated to this journey you are about to go on. Write down your schedule and mark down your progress. This will also help you go back and track your performance, as well as see where you have slipped up – giving you the ability to identify opportunities for improvement in the future.

If you rather prefer to keep things digital, then try out a couple of intermittent fasting apps. You would be surprised at how many there are. Take a look at some – they are available on both Google Play Store and Apple Store. Consider the user reviews. Then decide on an app that you like – and try to use it every day to help you keep track of your journey.

LIFE is currently one of the top-rated apps used for this purpose. It gives you the ability to record data for any type of intermittent fasting method that you would like to follow. You can easily adjust your schedule, and the app will even tell you when your body is expected to be in the ketosis phase. To keep you inspired and motivated, the app also allows you to join groups of other people who are on the same journey as you are.

BodyFast

https://play.google.com/store/apps/details?id=com.bodyfast&hl=en

Bodyfast app helps you to shed pounds fast in a healthful way. After a brief time, you will see the effects. The bottom for this intermittent fasting is you are taking a smash from ingesting in various periods. As an amateur, you'll examine intermittent fasting quickly, as an expert, you'll get precious aid. The Bodyfast app calculates your optimum fasting plan primarily based on your goals. Additional weekly demanding situations for a more fit life lead you to fulfilment.

MyFast

https://play.google.com/store/apps/details?id=com.prestigeworldwide.myfast&hl=en

Myfast fast allows you to understand intermittent fasting and could help you absolutely control your fasting schedule. You will stay on track to losing weight and enhancing your health.

Vora

https://play.google.com/store/apps/details?id=com.fastapp&hl=en

Vora aids in voraciously gulping a large meal after fasting, Vora is a cloud-based rapid tracker app where you may generate, edit, and cancel your fasts. Vora permits any fasting software to be used as long as you want Vora to track it for you.

Zero

https://play.google.com/store/apps/details?id=com.zerofasting.zero&hl=en

Zero is an easy fasting tracker used for custom, intermittent, and circadian rhythm fasting. Ensure that the favorite fasting protocol is picked, and zero will show your ongoing development for your Apple or iPhone watch. For the entire manipulate, export your report to a spreadsheet.

FastHabit

https://apps.apple.com/us/app/fasthabit-intermittent-fasting/id974978016

Fasthabit helps you start and remain regular with intermittent fasting. Set your duration for fasting, ensure that you log in every day and use advanced functions like multi-day, statistics export, calendar perspectives, apple watch integration, fitness and weight tracking app syncing and reminders are fasting to track your development and boost up your results.

Track Your Fast

https://play.google.com/store/apps/details?id=com.appsbybrent.trackyourfast&hl=en

Whether or not you've been intermittent fasting for years or have begun on your journey, track your fast app expedites you to record periods of fasting, so you can maximise fat loss by improving your consistency. Track your fast app comes with a free notification widget so that you can test your progress without ever having to release your telephone!

CHAPTER 10: LIST OF SHORT AND UNIQUE RECIPES FOR DIET

For this recipe portion, I've mixed the Keto Diet in with our attempts for Intermittent Fasting because the two pairs so easily. Typically, the Keto Diet is divided into the following nutritional percentages: around 70% of calories from fat, around 20% of calories from protein (a moderate amount), and no more than 10% of calories from carbohydrates.

The main focus of the Keto Diet is to remove excess carbohydrates from one's diet to enable the increased production of ketones in the body, which are essentially molecules that produce fuel for the individual. With less glucose, or blood sugar, in the body (resulting from that restriction of carbohydrates), the liver breaks down fat cells and produces ketones instead. Therefore, the body runs mostly off fat and burns fat more consistently because fat becomes **essential** for its ability to breakdown into ketones (a.k.a.—energy for brain and body).

With this increased production of ketones, the body becomes slimmer and fit, less bulked with fat, less sugar-crazed, and more energised even if the individual is intermittently fasting as well. In fact, Intermittent Fasting increases the body's production of ketones differently (by producing ketosis, a fruitful metabolic state), so the two pair well together in that ketonic connection.

As a general warning, just like with Intermittent Fasting, some body types will not do well with this type of metabolic shift. If you are diabetic, breastfeeding, or taking medication for high blood pressure and you still want to attempt Intermittent Fasting, I do not recommend adding the Keto Diet to the mix. For the rest of my readers, this section should help to solidify those weight loss and lifestyle goals in no time.

Low-carb breakfasts might seem counter-intuitive, but they're not only just possible! They're also delicious, nutritious, and packed with productive energy. Whichever of the two recipes below you choose, your mornings are sure to give you exactly the boost you need, and if you need more options, there are surely other sources at your disposal.

Frittata with Spinach and Mushrooms

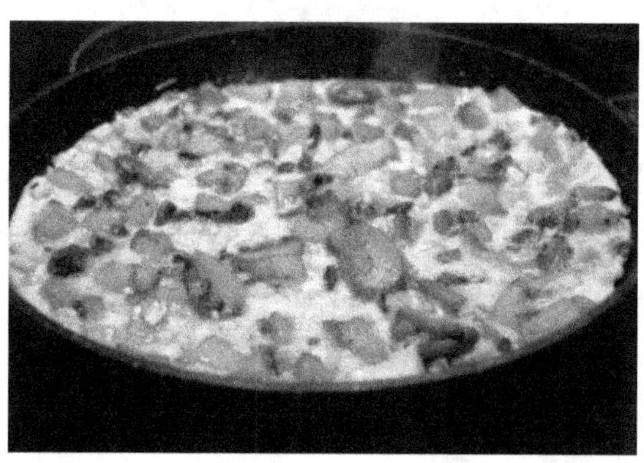

Tasty, simple, and packed with nutrition, this breakfast is best for sharing with a group of people (so there are no leftovers!) to get your day started.

This recipe needs 10 minutes of prep and about 35 minutes of cooking. It will make 4 helpings.

Fat—59 g

Protein—27 g

Net Carbs—4.1 g

Calories—661

What to Use:

Butter (2 tablespoons)

Bacon (6 ounces, coarsely diced)

Spinach (8 ounces)

Eggs (8, large-sized)

Heavy Cream (1 cup)

Shredded Cheese (6 ounces)

Salt & Pepper (to taste)

What to Do:

Start by heating the oven to 350 degrees while bringing the 2 tablespoons of butter to medium heat in a frying pan on the stovetop.

When heated, add bacon to pan and cook until desired crispiness. Then add the spinach and stir together until soft. Remove both from pan and drain the fat. Set to the side for now.

In a separate medium-sized bowl, combine the eggs and cream. Once whisked together, grease a 9x9 baking dish and pour the mixture in.

Stir in bacon, spinach, and any shredded cheese. Put dish and mixture in the oven.

Bake 30 minutes until perfectly browned.

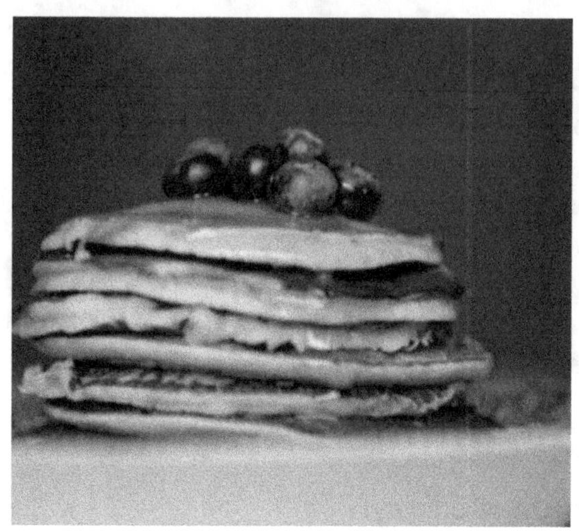

"How do you make low-carb pancakes?!" you might be asking yourself, and the answer is just within reach! These pancakes have a unique flavor, but they're nutritionally amazing and great for starting your day.

This recipe needs 5-10 minutes of prep and about 20 minutes of cooking. It will make 4 helpings.

Fat—39 g

Protein—13 g

Net Carbs—5 g

Calories—425

What to Use:

Eggs (4, large-sized)

Cottage Cheese (7 ounces)

Psyllium Husk Powder (1 tablespoon)

Butter or Coconut Oil (2 ounces)

Berries (0.5 cup, for topping)

What to Do:

In a medium-sized mixing bowl, stir together the first three ingredients and let sit. After about 10 minutes, the mixture should be perfectly thickened.

Grab a large-sized non-stick skillet and heat butter or coconut oil until melted. Portion out 0.5-cup scoops of the batter onto the skillet and cook 4 minutes on each side until done.

Prepare berries as desired (sliced or whole, etc.), and top finished pancakes with them for a delightful boost of sweetness

Lunch

For lunch, let's not do something too big or too packed with sugar. Salads, half-wraps, stir-fries, and chicken salads will do just fine! Regardless of your tastes, there should be something to suit your pallet in this section. Given your goals and vision for Intermittent Fasting, you're bound to see progress with these recipes in no time.

Curry Chicken Half-Wraps

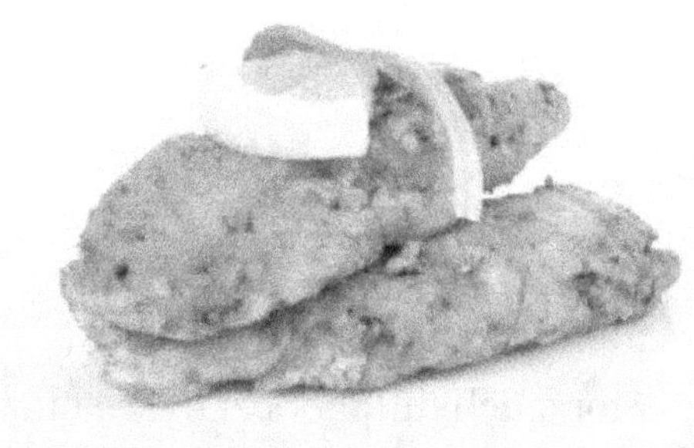

With a little effort, these half-wraps can be substituted for lettuce wraps, but they're just as delicious either way! Have as many as you need to keep that energy up throughout your day. There is a little less fat in this recipe than there could be, but you can correct that (as you like) by adding a little more cream as your garnish, or you could add a sprinkle of feta cheese on top, too.

This recipe needs 5 minutes of prep and about 20 minutes of cooking. It will make 2 helpings.

Fat—36.4 g

Protein—50.9 g

Net Carbs—7.2 g

Calories—554

What to Use:

Chicken Thighs (1 pound, boneless & skinless)

Onion (0.25 cup, minced)

Garlic (2 cloves, minced)

Curry Powder (2 teaspoons)

Salt (1.5 teaspoons)

Butter (3 tablespoons)

Cauliflower Rice (1 cup)

Low-Carb Wraps (cut into halves)

Or lettuce leaves

Yogurt or Sour Cream (0.25 cup, for garnish)

What to Do:

Start by preparing your chicken thighs; cut them into one-inch pieces.

Take a large-sized skillet and heat 2 of the 3 tablespoons of butter on the skillet at medium heat. Add onion and cook till soft and browned.

Stir in chicken pieces, garlic, and salt. Cook for about 10 minutes.

Stir in the last tablespoon of butter, curry powder, and cauliflower rice. Cook about 5 minutes longer.

Serve in lettuce leaves or half-wraps, and top with a scoop of cream!

Enjoy.

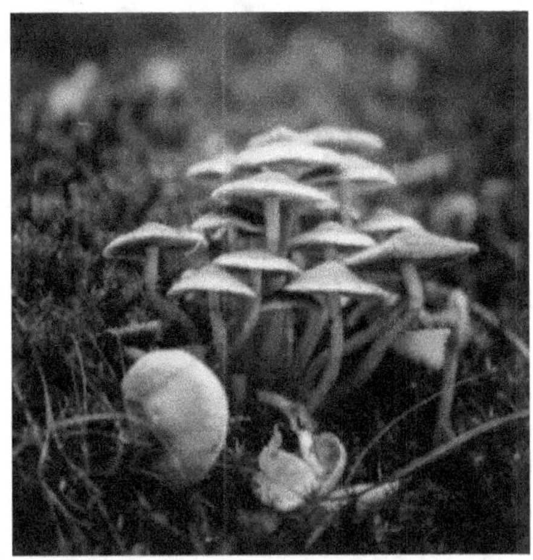

With a modest side-salad, this entrée is both elegant and appropriately filling. You'll want to bring it out when friends come around—or even for date night! The possibilities are endless.

This recipe needs 10 minutes of prep and about 10 minutes of cooking. It will make 2 helpings.

Fat—14 g

Protein—15 g

Net Carbs—8.4 g

Calories—257

What to Use:

Bacon (4 slices, cut into half-inch pieces)

Mushrooms (2 cups, halved; your choice)

Salt (0.5 teaspoon)

Thyme (2 sprigs fresh herb, destemmed)

Garlic (3 cloves, minced)

Greens (2 cups; your choice)

Salad Dressing (0.25 cup; your choice)

What to Do:

Assemble the side-salad quickly by taking your choice of greens and sprinkling on a bit of dressing. Set aside or place in the refrigerator for just a few moments.

Take a large-sized skillet and bring to medium heat. Add bacon and cook until desired crispiness is reached. Stir in mushrooms and bring to browned color.

Stir in salt, thyme leaves, and garlic. Cook 5 minutes then serve hot alongside your salad.

Easy Chicken Salad

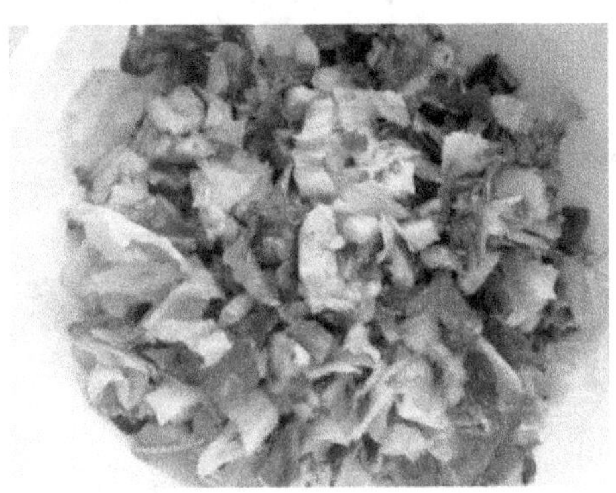

With a bread substitute of your choosing or over greens, this chicken salad will do just the trick. It even adds an interesting flavour spin on the traditional chicken salad that you can either appreciate or alter to your preferences. There is a little less fat in this recipe than what is typical of the Keto Diet, and you can correct that (for your liking) by adding more mayo or a bit of cheese to your salad as well.

This recipe needs 1 hour and 30 minutes of prep and about 15 minutes of cooking. It will make 6 helpings.

Fat—19 g

Protein—24.8 g

Net Carbs—1.1 g

Calories—279

What to Use:

Chicken Breast (1.5 pound)

Celery (3 stalks, sliced)

Mayo (0.5 cup)

Brown Mustard (2 teaspoons)

Salt (0.5 teaspoon)

Dill (2 tablespoons, fresh & chopped)

Pecans (0.25 cup, chopped)

What to Do:

Heat the oven to 425 degrees and line a baking sheet with parchment paper, aluminum foil, or baking spray.

Add chicken breast and cook until done throughout. This will take about 15 minutes.

Cool the breast completely. This can take anywhere from 10-30 minutes. Once cooled, cut into bite-size pieces.

Take a large-sized bowl and stir everything except the dill and pecans together.

Cover and chill about 1 hour before adding in dill and pecans. Serve cold.

Parmesan Bacon-Asparagus Roll-Ups

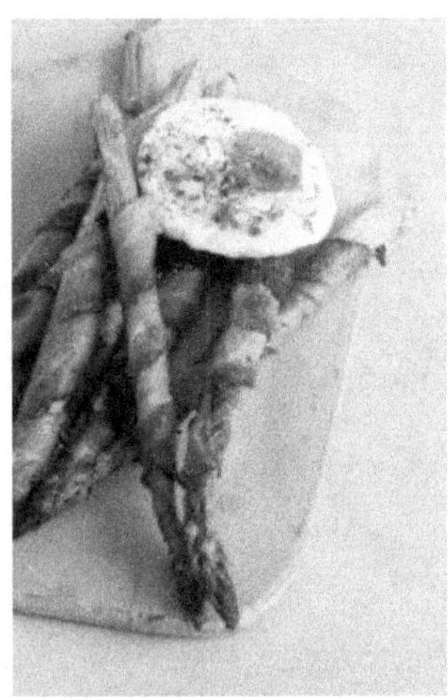

With the perfect touches of sweetness from the maple-flavoured syrup and char from the baking process, these roll-ups are either the best treat ever or the perfect small meal. Enjoy as many as you like. If you need more protein than is provided in this recipe, an easy fix would be to make a chicken breast on the side. The flavour boost would be incredible with that addition, too!

This recipe needs 15 minutes of prep and about 40 minutes of cooking. It will make 2 helpings.

Fat—23 g

Protein—7 g

Net Carbs—10.8 g

Calories—257

What to Use:

Maple-Flavoured Syrup (0.5 cup)

Butter (0.5 cup)

Salt (0.5 teaspoon)

Black Pepper (0.25 teaspoon)

Asparagus (2 pounds, washed & ends removed)

Bacon (8 slices, thick bacon)

Parmesan (2 tablespoons + 2 teaspoons, grated)

What to Do:

Start by preheating oven to 425 degrees.

Then, grab a small-sized pot and bring it to medium-low heat on the stove top. Add syrup, butter, salt, and pepper. Whisk together until smooth and heated through. Set aside for later.

Divide your 2 pounds of asparagus into 8 equal-sized groups. Wrap each group with a strip of bacon and secure the ends with toothpicks, as needed.

Line greased baking sheet with asparagus/bacon bundles then pour over with syrup mixture and half the parmesan.

Bake in the oven for 30 minutes. Then, switch to broil and bring the rack to the top shelf of the oven.

Broil 2 minutes until crispy and partially-charred.

Serve with toothpicks removed and enjoy!

For dinner tonight, let's try something simple. No need for a bunch of different devices or kitchen appliances. No need for fancy spices and hours upon hours of prep. These dinner recipes are easy and accessible, yet they don't sacrifice any bit of flavour potential. They're bound to give your taste buds a delight while providing all the energy you need and fill you up for your next stint of fasting.

Single-Pan Fajita Steak

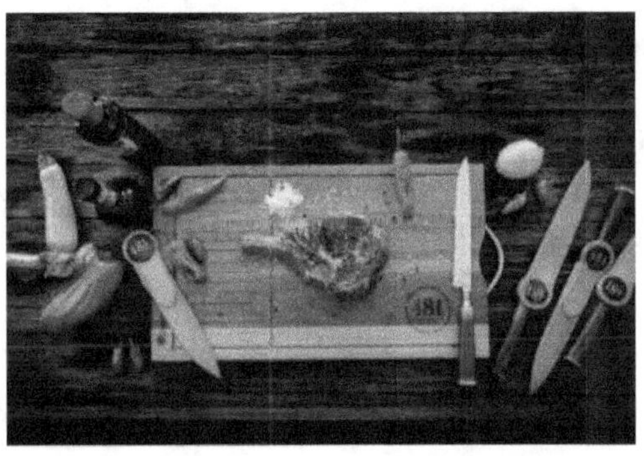

With just one sheet pan, this recipe comes together quickly and packs quite the punch for flavour! Combine it with low-carb tortillas of your choosing, eat over greens, or munch as-is. This dish is sure to please.

This recipe needs 5 minutes of prep and about 15 minutes of cooking. It will make 5 helpings.

Fat—33 g

Protein—31 g

Net Carbs—5 g

Calories—440

What to Use:

Garlic (2 cloves, minced)

Onion (1 medium-sized, sliced thinly)

Chili Powder (1 teaspoon)

Cumin (1 tablespoon)

Salt & Pepper (to taste)

Coconut Oil (0.25 cup)

Lime (1, juiced & zested)

Lemon (1, juiced & zested)

Steak (1 pound, sliced into strips)

Red Pepper (1 large-sized, sliced into strips)

Yellow Pepper (1 large-sized, sliced into strips)

What to Do:

Prepare the meat and vegetables and then stir all ingredients together on a lined or greased baking sheet.

Preheat oven to 350 degrees then bake for 15 minutes. Half-way through the process, stir the mixture well.

Serve with an extra sprinkle of lime juice.

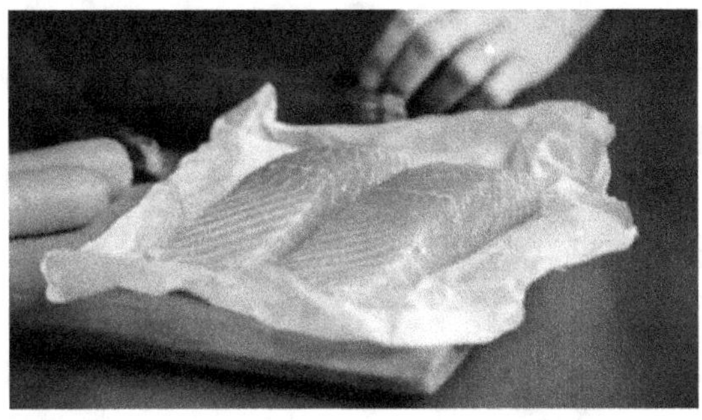

With just a handful of ingredients and a few simple steps, this recipe is gloriously easy and even more delicious than you could ever imagine. Trust me. Try it.

This recipe needs 5 minutes of prep and about 25 minutes of cooking. It will make 6 helpings.

Fat—30 g

Protein—54 g

Net Carbs—2 g

Calories—494

What to Use:

Olive Oil (2 tablespoons)

Salmon Fillets (3, 6-ounce fillets)

Garlic (2 cloves, minced)

Light Cream (1 cup)

Cream Cheese (1 ounce)

Capers (2 tablespoons)

Lemon Juice (1 tablespoon)

Dill (2 teaspoons, fresh OR 1 tablespoon, dried)

Parmesan Cheese (2 tablespoons, grated)

What to Do:

Grab a medium-sized skillet and heat the oil to start. Add the salmon fillets once heated through and cook 5 minutes on each side.

Set fish aside to get the sauce together.

In that same pan, add garlic and cook on medium heat for 2 minutes. Add cream, cream cheese, lemon juice, and capers. Simmer for 5 minutes or until thickened.

Once thickening begins, return salmon to pan and spoon the sauce over each of the fillets.

On low heat now, bring the salmon to the appropriate temperature. Garnish with dill and parmesan and serve!

Hard-Boiled Eggs

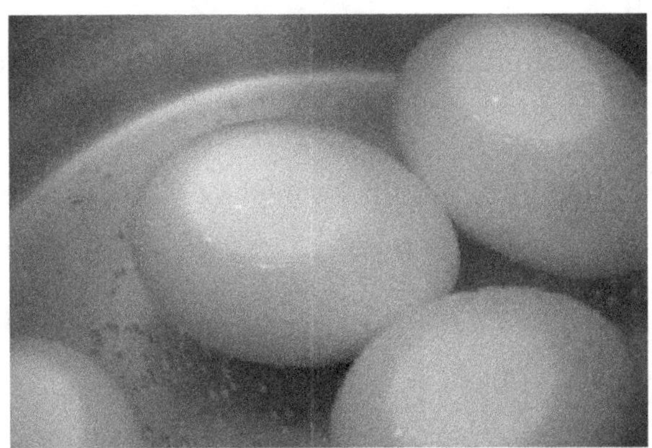

The most basic and reliable snack of all time is possibly the hard-boiled egg. With the right sprinkle of salt and pepper on top, it's hard to go wrong.

This recipe needs 5-10 minutes of cooking. It will make 4 helpings.

Fat—29 g

Protein—11 g

Net Carbs—1 g

Calories—316

What to Use:

Eggs (8, large-sized)

Salt & Pepper (to taste)

What to Do:

Take a small-sized pot and fill it ¾ of the way with water. Bring to boil.

Carefully, lay the eggs into the water and boil anywhere from 5-10 minutes. 5 minutes makes a softer egg, while 10 makes a firm and hard-boiled egg.

Serve with topping of salt & pepper or otherwise.

Unforgettable Spaghetti Squash

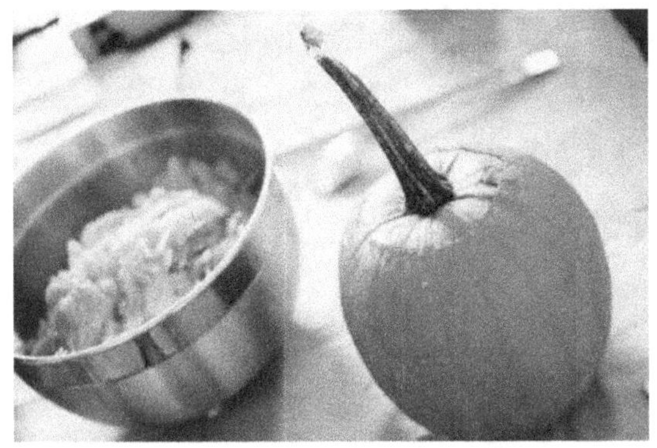

If you're like me and somewhat picky with winter squash, you're bound to be as amazed as I was when you try this spaghetti squash recipe. No pasta required, given the unique nature of this squash, and with the cheese and garlic topping, even picky eaters will surprise themselves by how much they like it. There's a little less protein in this meal than there could be, but you can boost your version by adding a little meat (try chorizo or bacon!) into the mix or by compensating through another snack or meal in the day instead.

This recipe needs 10 minutes of prep and about 1 hour of cooking. It will make 4 helpings.

Fat—24.4 g

Protein—8 g

Net Carbs—3.1 g

Calories—274

What to Use:

Spaghetti Squash (1 medium-sized OR equivalent of 3 pounds)

Garlic (3 cloves, minced)

Olive Oil (1 teaspoon)

Spinach (half-pound, chopped)

Heavy Cream (0.5 cup)

Parmesan Cheese (0.5 cup)

Salt & Pepper (to taste)

Mozzarella (grated for topping)

What to Do:

First, preheat the oven to 400 degrees.

Prepare the spaghetti squash by cutting it in half (lengthwise) and pulling out any seeds.

Line a baking sheet or grease it and lay spaghetti squash with the cut side down on the sheet. Roast 30-40 minutes until easily stabbed through with a fork.

Meanwhile, prepare the sauce. In a medium-sized pot, heat olive oil and garlic for no more than 5 minutes. Stir in spinach, cream, and parmesan in turn.

Season with salt and pepper and set aside.

When squash has finished roasting, pull it out from oven and begin to pull apart the strands of the squash itself (its name should make sense to you now if it didn't already!).

With the squash threads freed, pour the cheese mixture onto the squash and into the inner "boat" part. Top with extra parmesan and mozzarella, as desired, then bake at 350 degrees for 20 additional minutes.

At the last second, switch oven to broil and bring cheese to a beautiful browned color. Enjoy hot!

CHAPTER 11: CASE STUDIES

Case study 1

When it comes to learning more about specific types of diet plans and lifestyle habits, it is always important to take a look at the scientific research behind such programs. With this in mind, the same applies to those who are interested in taking on an intermittent fasting plan – whether it is to lose weight or to build muscle mass or to enjoy a healthy way of living simply and to experience the benefits. If you are interested in intermittent fasting, be sure to first take a good look at the scientific evidence behind this eating plan. Do not only consider the potential benefits that intermittent fasting might have for you, but also consider the possible side-effects and downsides that may apply to those who are following a diet that is based on intermittent fasting.

Many scientific studies have been done on intermittent fasting, which can help you determine the efficiency and safety of this particular diet program. In this chapter, I would like to go over a few of the previous studies that have been conducted.

"Daily fasting works for weight loss, finds the report on 16:8 diet."

The University of Illinois at Chicago published the results of a recent study they conduct, titled Daily fasting works for weight loss, finds the report on 16:8 diet. The study was officially published on ScienceDaily on the 18th of June, 2018.

The study focused on obtaining data relevant to the effects of intermittent fasting on the body weight of individuals who are obese. There was a total of 23 volunteers who participated in the study. All of the volunteers were obese, with a BMI that measured 35 or higher. The average age of the participants was about 45.

During the study, the participants were asked to consume their meals between 10 am in the morning and 6 pm at night During the rest of the day, the participant was asked to undergo a fast – where they were not allowed to consume any type of food or beverages, except for water and selected beverages that do not contain calories. This particular study lasted for a total of 12 weeks.

Several benefits were noted by the scientists who were involved in the study. The results that were obtained in this study were compared to results from a previous study that also focused on the effects of fasting on obesity and body weight, but that previous study did not implement time-restricted fasting protocols.

In particular, this study found that weight loss was much more significant among those individuals who followed an intermittent fasting diet plan. Calorie consumption was also reduced by a statistically significant level. In addition to the weight-related benefits, it was also found that the study participants experienced an improvement in their blood pressure levels. With obesity being linked to high blood pressure – and this condition, in turn, associated with a range of adverse effects in the body, including blood vessel damage, this is certainly a benefit that needs to be noted.

The average participant in this particular study was found to consume 350 calories less than they did before they started to follow the intermittent fasting diet that was presented to them by the researchers involved in the study. Additionally, the individuals involved in the study were also found to lose an average of 3% of their total body weight. Additionally, systolic blood pressure levels were decreased by an average of seven millimeters per mercury, or mm Hg.

Scientists involved in the study concluded by saying that the obese population should know that there are ways that they can lose weight effectively without the need for excessively starving themselves, without having to count calories to the last digit, and without the need to eliminate all of the most tasteful foods that they are used to consuming.

It should be noted that results in this particular study on intermittent fasting and the diet's effect on weight loss had similar results compared to the previous studies that focused on fasting in general in terms of insulin resistance, cholesterol regulation, and fat mass. Still, this holds important evidence that intermittent fasting can be a good tool in a person's weight loss strategy.

Case study 2

"Intermittent fasting interventions for the treatment of overweight and obesity in adults."

A study conducted scientists at the University of Glasgow in the United Kingdom, published on the 1st of February 2018, looked at how intermittent fasting could be utilised as an intervention in the treatment of excessive weight among adults in the local region. The study was conducted in such a way to compare the results obtained with intermittent fasting to the results that can be achieved through no treatment, as well as through more traditional means of treating obesity in adult patients.

All of the patients who were part of the study had a BMI that was more than 25, which classifies them as being overweight. A large number of the study participants were obese as well, which means their BMI was higher than 30. All of the participants were over the age of 18 at the time of the study.

Each patient who participated in the study were provided with a diet plan that they had to follow. On intermittent fasting days, the patient was advised to consume a diet that resulted in less than 800 kcal in total consumption per day. The study lasted for 12 weeks in total to ensure adequate time for results to be achieved, as it is known that appropriate weight loss results with any changes in diet can take a while.

The most significant results noted by this study were the reduction in the body weight of the participants who were involved in the intermittent fasting diet. In addition to these primary outcomes of the study, there were several secondary outcomes that the scientists who were involved in the study noted as well.

The secondary outcomes presented by the study was divided into multiple groups, and consists of:

- Anthropometric outcomes: Participants had a lower BMI at the end of the study and smaller waist circumference. Fat mass and fat-free mass were also reduced significantly, compared to the other studies that were compared to the results obtained from the intermittent fasting programs.

- Cardio-metabolic outcomes: Blood glucose levels were improved, along with insulin levels. The study also noted statistically significant improvements in the blood pressure levels of patients who participated in the intermittent fasting program. Lipoprotein profiles had also improved.

It should be noted that some results obtained in the intermittent fasting study were very similar to the results that were obtained in the other studies that these results were compared to.

In the end, this is yet another study that provides evidence of the effective results that intermittent fasting can provide a person with if they follow through on the particular plan that has been developed for them. Dedication and patience are two key factors to ensure the individual following this type of diet is able to achieve success and reach the goals they have set out for themselves.

CHAPTER 12: COMMON QUESTIONS

Can I drink coffee while I am fasting?

Coffee is a beverage that millions of people enjoy each and every day. This is why many people are concerned that they might have to give up their cup of coffee that they enjoy so much each morning if they are going to start following an intermittent fasting plan – the majority of these plans will tell you to sustain from eating until later in the afternoon and to skip on breakfast for a boost in benefits.

Fortunately, there is no need to worry if you are planning to implement intermittent fasting into your diet – and would still like to have a cup or two of coffee in the morning. There is, however, one particular factor that you do need to note here. If you want to have a cup of coffee after waking up and your intermittent fasting plan demands that you continue with your fasting window in the morning, then it means no sugar and no milk for you. While some people have noted that it is okay to add one splash of milk to your coffee while fasting, this is usually not recommended if you are serious about losing weight while you are following an intermittent fasting plan.

Coffee can actually be a great addition to your diet plan and be a good boost for getting through that last period of fasting. When you opt for a cup of coffee in the morning, you will get an energy boost – and since the caffeine in coffee may provide you with benefits for as long as six hours, you can easily glide on these effects until the time comes to break your fasting period.

Coffee has also been shown to speed up metabolism, which is great for anyone looking to lose weight. You'll end up burning even more fat.

Additionally, coffee will help to keep your mind sharp during the morning and avoid those dreadful times when brain fog hits you because you are running on empty.

There is another benefit that should be noted in terms of having a cup of coffee for breakfast, instead of indulging in a big breakfast. This particular benefit comes in handy for those who are looking to work out while they are still fasting – many people prefer a morning workout, after all. There are some people who follow an intermittent fasting plan that finds they do not have the same level of energy while working out compared to eating a good breakfast before they go out and hit the gym. When you drink some coffee, you'll get a boost in both physical performances, and cognitive function – both of these are crucial for a good workout in the gym.

Should I break my fast with a big or small meal?

Another popular question that people tend to ask when it comes to intermittent fasting is how exactly they should break their fast. The opinions in regards to breaking a fasting window while following an intermittent fasting program is mixed. Some suggest that you break the fast with a big meal that is packed with calories to load your body with protein and other essential nutrients, while others suggest that you start out simple and small, and then gradually work up to that big meal.

There really isn't a single perfect answer to this question, but it should be taken into account that when breaking a fast, the body is still in a fat burning mode. When you hit your body with too many calories at once, you can switch off this mode and experience less of the benefits that you are expecting from your intermittent fasting plan.

Thus, it is generally not considered a good idea to break your fast with a meal that is considered loaded in calories. I personally find that it is much more convenient to start things out slowly. Perhaps break that fasting period with a green salad, or perhaps some Greek yogurt. There are many options that can help to satisfy the hunger you have built up during the fast, offer you a series of healthy and essential nutrients, but without causing your metabolism to shut down.

After the fast has been broken and you have had your first meal, plan for a second and a third meal as well. Be sure that these meals will also be nutritious and healthy. I enjoy a big meal that makes up most of the calories I should consume daily by the end of the day. Some might prefer this "big meal" to happen in between their first and third meal – this way, they can start their eating cycle and end the cycle with something small. This would also help to reduce the number of calories you should consume just before you go to bed.

If you are not sure which one you prefer, be sure to consider the various meal plan examples that I have shared with you in this book. You'll find a couple of different meal plans spread out throughout this book – they are all great for those who are starting out without knowing which type of meal plan they would like to implement with their intermittent fasting program.

A good idea would also be to experiment with different options. Try to make the second meal of the eating period your big meal of the day. See how your body reacts. You might also try the first and the final meal of the day – make these your big meals. Really observe how you feel with each of these options. You'll eventually start to notice that your body reacts better to one of these particular options – or perhaps spreading out your calories equally. When you find the right option, continue with it.

How do I cope with my hunger during the fasting window?

When you are starting out with intermittent fasting for the first time and you are used to eating three or more meals a day, along with some snacking in-between, then there really is no doubt that for the initial period of intermittent fasting, you will experience hunger and some cravings. This is something that most people struggle with – and it is an issue that often causes people to give up on intermittent fasting and either return to their usual way of eating or turn to another type of diet to help them possibly lose the excess weight that is causing them concern.

The key to success in terms of coping with hunger when starting with

an intermittent fasting program really is patience. You will need to have patience when it comes to feeling the effects of this diet come into play. It will take some time, but when you push through these hunger strikes, then you will start to notice the cravings become fewer and fewer as the days go by. Instead of experiencing cravings for candy and other unhealthy foods, you will start to experience hunger – this is a good thing, so do not think of the hunger as a bad thing that is striking you at the most unpleasant times.

Since you are not craving unhealthy foods, you will be less likely to start searching for donuts and candy bars to snack on. You'll also find that it is easier to push through until you reach the time where you can have your first meal.

If you do feel that you are unable to cope anymore and those last few hours simply seem too far away, then have sparkling water. This will help to make your stomach feel full for a little while – in turn, and you will find that it becomes much easier to last for an hour or two more in order to reach the time when you can finally break your fast.

How will I train if I am running empty on food?

While coping with hunger is one thing that people struggle with when they are following an intermittent fasting plan, another issue that some also find is that they are not sure how they will continue with their training regimen once they start to follow this type of program. The obvious idea behind intermittent fasting is that you would find yourself running low on food just in the nick of time when you decide to hit the gym – this means you do not have an adequate source of fuel to give you that energy you need to push through the entire session.

In reality, some people actually find that they are able to train more efficiently when their stomach is not full. There are also many who have claimed training during a fasting period is more beneficial – and that it is sometimes even easier.

If you do feel that you are unable to get through that upcoming training session because you feel "empty" and out of energy, then perhaps consider opting for a cup of coffee – no milk or sugar, however. The coffee will give you the boost you need to get through the entire session and may even give you some energy afterward to last until the time at which you can break the fast.

Keep in mind that when training on an empty stomach, your body will not have food to turn to in order to generate energy. In turn, this also means that your body will start to turn to the fat storages within your body in order to generate the energy that you need to continue running on that treadmill or to continue pushing those weights. This, in turn, also means fat is burnt faster and much more effectively.

Is it okay to cheat now-and-then?

When it comes to intermittent fasting for weight loss, people are usually inclined to follow a specific meal plan and diet that will give them guidance on what they can eat during the periods that they are allowed to consume calories. In the majority of cases, diets will be somewhat restricted – they will usually include healthy foods that are relatively low in carbohydrates while being high in protein and other essential nutrients.

The healthy meals will surely make you feel great, but there is no shame in wanting to have a "cheat" snack or even a cheat meal now-and-then. The big question now is whether or not it is okay for you to have a cheat day, or even just a cheat snack or treat.

In reality, having a "cheat" day will not do you a lot of harm in terms of your weight loss results – the important part here is to ensure that this does not happen every day. Try to limit yourself to a cheat once a week at most. Perhaps grab a bar of chocolate from your local supermarket or, if you really want to go bigger, get your family to agree to dinner at a local restaurant.

When you do have a cheat day or meal, it is important that you take the calories consumed while 'cheating' into account. This number of calories you will have to make up for the next day – this way, you'll continue to experience the benefits of the diet.

Consider the number of calories you went over your daily limit today – perhaps that bar of chocolate added another 150 calories to your day.

The next day, be sure to reduce your calorie consumption to make up for the excess in calories that you decided to have the previous day.

CONCLUSION

I hope this book helped you understand the basics of occasional fasting and the benefits that this diet will bring into your life. By practicing occasionally fasting while you are fit, without having to adhere to strict diets that can be harmful to your health, you will succeed in reducing weight and be in the best form of your life.

Understanding the principles of occasional fasting, will not only help to reduce your weight, but it will also contribute to the strengthening of your mental health by training your brain to be durable and to resist food in moments that are meant for fasting. This way you will become a stronger person. But the psyche is not the only thing that will be strengthened. Who does not want strong and well-shaped muscles? Well, occasional fasting will help in creating this. You must be wondering how can something that deprives you of food, helps you build muscle when you know that building muscle requires more calorie intake. Well, this is not the case. Basically, intermittent fasting will teach you to appreciate food and to refer to a healthy diet that will become part of your everyday life. With the right combination of fat, carbohydrates, protein, fresh fruits and vegetables, you will able to create meals that the body needs on the days of not fasting.

The next step is to list all the various methods of intermittent fasting once more, to help you choose the one that will best suit your lifestyle and daily responsibilities, and gradually start to change your life and take care of your health forever. Of course, do not be alarmed if you are suddenly unable to endure the whole fasting period. Allow your body some time to get used to this way of eating, and over time you will be able to lengthen the time for fasting. Combine some simple exercises to increase the burning of fat from your body, or prepare your own exercise plan that will fit your fitness level. But, try not to forget the recommendations given in the book of the combination of the intensity of exercise on the days when you are fasting and the days when you are not fasting.

It is important to plan exercise days wells. If you practice high-intensity workouts on the fasting day, you will feel exhausted, and your muscles will be under a lot of stress, which is not good when you are trying to shape and enhance. Also, to get those well established and toned muscles, drink plenty of water (at least eight glasses, but really this is the minimum amount we need) and remember to combine protein, carbohydrates, and fat before and after training to help your muscles grow. Take the recommendations for gradual entry into the process of fasting and become one step closer to changing your whole life and becoming happier and satisfied with your visual appearance and health.

Thank you for choosing this book. Make sure to **leave an honest review on Amazon** if you wish, I'd like to know what you think!